Statistics for Biology and Health

Series Editors:
M. Gail
K. Krickeberg
J. Samet
A. Tsiatis
W. Wong

Statistics for Biology and Health

Aalen/Borgan/Gjessing: Survival and Event History Analysis: A Process Point of View
Bacchieri/Cioppa: Fundamentals of Clinical Research
Borchers/Buckland/Zucchini: Estimating Animal Abundance: Closed Populations
Burzykowski/Molenberghs/Buyse: The Evaluation of Surrogate Endpoints
Duchateau/Janssen: The Frailty Model
Everitt/Rabe-Hesketh: Analyzing Medical Data Using S-PLUS
Ewens/Grant: Statistical Methods in Bioinformatics: An Introduction, 2nd ed.
Gentleman/Carey/Huber/Irizarry/Dudoit: Bioinformatics and Computational Biology
    Solutions Using R and Bioconductor
Hougaard: Analysis of Multivariate Survival Data
Keyfitz/Caswell: Applied Mathematical Demography, 3rd ed.
Klein/Moeschberger: Survival Analysis: Techniques for Censored and Truncated Data,
    2nd ed.
Kleinbaum/Klein: Survival Analysis: A Self-Learning Text, 2nd ed.
Kleinbaum/Klein: Logistic Regression: A Self-Learning Text, 2nd ed.
Lange: Mathematical and Statistical Methods for Genetic Analysis, 2nd ed.
Manton/Singer/Suzman: Forecasting the Health of Elderly Populations
Martinussen/Scheike: Dynamic Regression Models for Survival Data
Moyé: Multiple Analyses in Clinical Trials: Fundamentals for Investigators
Nielsen: Statistical Methods in Molecular Evolution
O'Quigley: Proportional Hazards Regression
Parmigiani/Garrett/Irizarry/Zeger: The Analysis of Gene Expression Data: Methods and
    Software
Proschan/LanWittes: Statistical Monitoring of Clinical Trials: A Unified Approach
Schlattmann: Medical Applications of Finite Mixture Models
Siegmund/Yakir: The Statistics of Gene Mapping
Simon/Korn/McShane/Radmacher/Wright/Zhao: Design and Analysis of DNA Microarray
    Investigations
Sorensen/Gianola: Likelihood, Bayesian, and MCMC Methods in Quantitative Genetics
Stallard/Manton/Cohen: Forecasting Product Liability Claims: Epidemiology and Modeling
    in the Manville Asbestos Case
Sun: The Statistical Analysis of Interval-censored Failure Time Data
Therneau/Grambsch: Modeling Survival Data: Extending the Cox Model
Ting: Dose Finding in Drug Development
Vittinghoff/Glidden/Shiboski/McCulloch: Regression Methods in Biostatistics: Linear,
    Logistic, Survival, and Repeated Measures Models
Wu/Ma/Casella: Statistical Genetics of Quantitative Traits: Linkage, Maps, and QTL
Zhang/Singer: Recursive Partitioning in the Health Sciences
Zuur/Ieno/Smith: Analysing Ecological Data

Peter Schlattmann

Medical Applications
of Finite Mixture Models

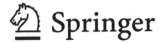 Springer

Dr. Peter Schlattmann
Department of Biostatistics
and Clinical Epidemiology
Charité Universitätsmedizin
Charitéplatz 1
10117 Berlin
Germany
peter.schlattmann@charite.de

Series Editors

M. Gail
National Cancer Institute
Rockville, MD 20892
USA

K. Krickeberg
Le Chatelet
F-63270 Manglieu
France

J. Samet
Department of Epidemiology
School of Public Health
Johns Hopkins University
615 Wolfe Street
Baltimore, MD 21205-2103
USA

A. Tsiatis
Department of Statistics
North Carolina State University
Raleigh, NC 27695
USA

W. Wong
Department of Statistics
Stanford University
Stanford, CA 94305-4065
USA

ISBN   978-3-642-08816-2   e-ISBN   978-3-540-68651-4
DOI 10.1007/978-3-540-68651-4

Cover design: WMXDesign GmbH, Heidelberg

Printed on acid-free paper

springer.com

Preface

Patients are not alike! This simple truth is often ignored in the analysis of medical data, since most of the time results are presented for the "average" patient. As a result, potential variability between patients is ignored when presenting, e.g., the results of a multiple linear regression model. In medicine there are more and more attempts to individualize therapy; thus, from the author's point of view biostatisticians should support these efforts. Therefore, one of the tasks of the statistician is to identify heterogeneity of patients and, if possible, to explain part of it with known explanatory covariates.

Finite mixture models may be used to aid this purpose. This book tries to show that there are a large range of applications. They include the analysis of gene expression data, pharmacokinetics, toxicology, and the determinants of beta-carotene plasma levels. Other examples include disease clustering, data from psychophysiology, and meta-analysis of published studies.

The book is intended as a resource for those interested in applying these methods. So the main focus is on introducing the ideas of finite mixture models and their ideas in various applications. The author hopes that this material is accessible to an audience with some quantitative background, such as (bio)statisticians, epidemiologists, pharmacokineticists, and interested physicians. The book assumes knowledge of statistics at an intermediate level; hence, familiarity with maximum likelihood estimation is assumed, since such methods are the basis for the statistical inference and estimation used throughout the book. The chapter on theory and algorithms is perhaps mathematically a bit more demanding. This chapter follows the idea to provide the necessary background in convex optimization necessary to understand the algorithms available for finite mixture models.

To provide easy to use software, the book is accompanied by the R (http://www.r-project.org) package CAMAN, which can be used to carry out many of the analyses performed in this book. The package and data sets available to the public may be found at http://www.charite.de/biometrie/schlattmann/book. Some of the analyses may also be performed with SAS. The corresponding code may also be found on the appropriate Web page.

I am grateful to many people who supported me in the preparation of the book. First of all, I would like to thank Dankmar Böhning, who introduced me to the field of finite mixture models and with whom I share a long-lasting collaboration. A part of the R package is based on our software C.A.MAN, which was published as standalone software. Also I would like to acknowledge the collaboration with Johannes Höhne, whose programming skills helped to create the R package. Further, I would like to thank my colleagues in the Department of Biostatistics and Clinical Epidemiology of Charité Universitätsmedizin Berlin for creating a stimulating environment. In particular I would like to thank Ekkehart Dietz, Katja Frieler, and Ben Rich for fruitful discussions. The head of the institute, Peter Martus, has given me continuous support over the years I have been employed there.

Also I would like to thank my former colleagues in the Department of Psychiatry and Psychotherapy for the fun to work with them and many insights into the thinking of practicing clinicians. I learned a lot from Heidi Danker-Hopfe, Maria Jockers-Scherübl, and Peter Neu.

My sincere thanks are given to the publisher, especially to Lilith Braun for her patience and support.

Finally, I am greatly indebted to my wife Kerstin Treichel for the continuous support and understanding during the preparation of this book.

Berlin, December 2008   *Peter Schlattmann*

Contents

Chapter 1
Overview of the Book

What can the reader expect from this book? The book intends to introduce the analysis of heterogeneity applied to medical data. A special tool for this kind of analysis are finite mixture models which may or may not be adjusted for covariates. Using examples from the medical literature, the book shows that these model may be useful in many medical applications. Possible applications range from early drug development to the meta-analysis of clinical studies. Others are disease mapping or the analysis of gene expression data, just to mention a few. Thus, another goal of the book is to provide easy-to-use software to make these methods available for the interested reader; therefore, a detailed description of how to use of the R package CAMAN is part of the book.

The book also handles some of the theory of finite mixture models. The understanding of this theory requires some knowledge of convex sets and convex optimization. The book attempts to provide the necessary mathematics needed for convex optimization which is difficult to find in the condensed form needed here.

The following pages give a general overview of the book.

Introduction

Chapter 2 illustrates the idea of heterogeneity in medicine. It starts with the observation that patients are not alike. In a therapeutic setting patients react differently to treatment regimes. Some patients do not respond to the treatment at all and others recover quickly under the treatment. This may depend on known factors such as genetic polymorphisms or age. This leads to the necessity to individualize therapy.

The clinical problem of individualizing therapy is related to the statistical problem of heterogeneity of treatment effects. Standard statistical models, such as linear regression, model the population average, which is the mean response of all individuals ("one size fits all"). Thus, the modest benefit observed in many clinical trials can be misleading because moderate average effects may be a mixture of substantial

P. Schlattmann, *Medical Applications of Finite Mixture Models*,
Statistics for Biology and Health, DOI: 10.1007/978-3-540-68651-4_1,
© Springer-Verlag Berlin Hiedelberg 2009

benefits for some, little, or no benefit for many and harm for a few. This is an indication of unobserved heterogeneity of patients which can be caused by an unknown covariate.

From a statistical point of view the total variability of the data is divided into two parts: The first part is the variability between individuals and the second part is residual or error variability. This leads to subject-specific or random effects models.

One such model is a finite mixture model. The basic ideas of this model are introduced in Chap. 2 for a hypothetical example from a clinical trial where only a moderate treatment benefit is observable. This example shows that in this hypothetical case the total population of patients consists of two subpopulations, one with considerable benefit and a larger proportion with little benefit. The corresponding proportions and average effects of each subpopulation need to be estimated from the data. With use of data from a study looking at determinants of beta-carotene plasma levels, a finite mixture model is applied to these data and it is shown how this model can be extended to include covariates.

An important part in drug therapy and development is the investigation of pharmacokinetics. Section 2.3 introduces the concept of population pharmacokinetics. This approach aims to model the relationship between physiologic function (both normal and disease altered) and pharmacokinetics while taking the interindividual variability in these relationships into account. Variability of the pharmacokinetic response between individuals may be caused by differences in absorption, elimination, and clearance. These differences may be due to genetic polymorphisms or factors such as age, gender, or reduced renal or hepatic function. However, these factors are often unknown, and as a result models are needed which can take unobserved covariates into account.

Analysis of Count Data

Chapter 3 describes the use of random effects models for count data. Here either parametric random effects models which assume a gamma distribution for the random effects or a finite mixture model is used.

The first part describes the analysis of count data without covariates. Here, data from a cohort study in northeast Thailand where the health status of 602 preschool children was checked every 2 weeks from June 1982 until September 1985 are analyzed. In this time period it was recorded how often the children showed symptoms of fever, cough, running nose, or all symptoms together.

It turns out that a simple Poisson distribution is not sufficient to model these data; thus, in Sect. 3.2 parametric mixture models and in Sect. 3.3 finite mixture models are fit to these data. A crucial point in fitting finite mixture models is the choice of the number of components k. Besides methods such as the likelihood ratio test, a nonparametric bootstrap method introduced by the author is applied. The analysis of the properties of this approach is one of the contributions of the author to the field of mixture models (Schlattmann 2003, 2005).

Section 3.5 analyses count data with covariates. This approach is developed using the Ames test as an example. This test simultaneously investigates the mutagenicity and the toxicity of a chemical. The Ames test uses a number of *Salmonella* strains with a preexisting mutation, which leaves the bacteria unable to synthesize the amino acid histidine and as result unable to grow and form colonies. New mutations can restore the gene's function and allow the cells to produce histidine. These newly mutated cells can grow in the absence of histidine and form colonies. This is cast into a regression problem for count data and the ideas of this regression model are developed starting from first principles. This leads to a standard Poisson regression model. Again, it turns out that this model does not describe the data well.

Thus, regression models based on the negative binomial distribution and covariate-adjusted mixture models are also applied to the data. These models provide a much better fit. To fit the covariate-adjusted finite mixture models, a newly developed algorithm is applied. This algorithm is developed in Chap. 4.

Theory and Algorithms

Chapter 4 introduces a new algorithm for covariate-adjusted mixture models in Sect. 4.6.4. It exploits the properties of the nonparametric maximum likelihood estimator of the mixing distribution. Since these results rely on basic results of convex analysis and optimization, these are introduced in Sect. 4.2.

Now we introduce a finite mixture model. Consider a sample $x_1, x_2, \ldots, x_n$ with

$$x_i \overset{\text{iid}}{\sim} f(x, P) \quad i = 1, \ldots, n, \tag{1.1}$$

$$f(x, P) = \sum_{j=1}^{k} p_j f(x, \lambda_j), \tag{1.2}$$

where p_j are the mixing weights, λ_j are the component parameters, k is the number of components, and $f(.)$ is a density. Estimation of the parameters of the mixing distribution P is predominantly done using maximum likelihood. We are interested in finding the maximum likelihood estimates of P which maximize the log likelihood function

$$\ell(P) = \log L(P) = \sum_{i=1}^{n} \log \sum_{j=1}^{k} p_j f(x_i, \lambda_j). \tag{1.3}$$

When fitting finite mixture models, we must distinguish two cases. The first is the *flexible* support size case, where no assumption about the number of components k is made in advance. This case is discussed in Sect. 4.3. In the *fixed* support size case the number of components k is assumed to be known. Here the unknown parameters are the mixing weights p_j and the parameters λ_j of the subpopulation. Section 4.4 discusses this case. Estimation of these models' parameters is usually achieved by application of the expectation maximization algorithm described in Sect. 4.4.3. This algorithm is well known to converge to local maxima depending on the starting values. For the case of finite mixtures without covariates, a globally convergent variant of the expectation maximization algorithm with gradient function update is available. It uses information based on the directional derivative of the likelihood function and exchanges the parameter which maximizes the gradient function to perform a vertex exchange step. This algorithm is described in Sect. 4.4.6.

Often the inclusion of covariates into the model is desirable and the researcher is interested in whether there is residual heterogeneity present after the inclusion of known covariates. This task may be cast into the framework of the covariate-adjusted mixture models described in Sect. 4.6. These fit into the framework of generalized linear mixed models. Section 4.6.1 describes first generalized linear models, then Sect. 4.6.2 shows how the expectation maximization algorithm for finite mixture models can be extended to adjust for covariates. Again, this algorithm converges to local maxima depending on the starting values. Hence, the expectation maximization algorithm is modified using a gradient update step. Here the maximum of the gradient function is difficult to find, e.g., by a bisection method. As an alternative we propose finding the maximum of the gradient function by simulated annealing. This procedure enables us to find the maximum of the gradient function even for a high-dimensional parameter space with many covariates. This new algorithm developed by the author is presented in detail in Sect. 4.6.4.

Finally, a case study demonstrates the use of the method for a population pharmacokinetic analysis of the analgesic drug Dipyrone in Sect. 4.7; it is demonstrated that the new algorithm provides an improved fit.

Disease Mapping and Cluster Investigations

Chapter 5 discusses the investigation of presumed clusters of disease. Frequently, such a cluster is presumed to be the result of a so-called focus. Thus, the distinction of generalized and focused clustering is introduced.

Investigations which seek to address "general clustering" determine whether or not cases are clustered anywhere in the study area, without a prior assumption about the location of a potential cluster. In contrast, tests addressing "focused" clustering assess whether cases are clustered around a prespecified source of hazard, which is frequently called a focus.

The first example in Sect. 5.2 investigates general clustering in the former East Germany, addressing the question whether there is an increase of childhood leukemia in the southeast or, more precisely, in the vicinity of the nuclear power plant at Rossendorf. To avoid a selection bias this investigation looked at the presence of general clustering, i.e., at the presence of heterogeneity of disease risk in the total region. In contrast to traditional methods such as percentile or probability maps, methods based on mixture models show a homogeneous distribution of disease risk.

Frequently, to assess the "nonrandomness" of a map, tests for autocorrelation or heterogeneity are applied. The latter accounts for the extra-Poisson variation frequently present in the homogeneous Poisson model. In Sect. 5.4 it is shown that overdispersion can be due either to autocorrelation or to heterogeneity of disease risk.

In contrast to general clustering, focused clustering studies investigate presumably raised incidence of disease in the vicinity of prespecified putative sources of increased risk. A frequently used test is the score test. It is shown that this test is a special case of Poisson regression. The assumption of a Poisson distribution for the data at hand is not necessarily true; hence, in Sect. 5.5.2 a robust version of the score is developed. This version implicitly allows for heterogeneity of disease risk. Section 5.5.3 develops a version of the score test which is based on the negative binomial distribution. This test thus explicitly allows for heterogeneity of disease risk. A case study in Sect. 5.6 analyses the association between leukemia in adults and the nuclear power plant at Krümmel. In this case the newly developed tests are applied to investigate the aforementioned association. Finally, Sect. 5.7 describes the mathematical basis for the newly developed score tests.

Modeling Heterogeneity in Psychophysiology

In Chap. 6 a new method is introduced to model spatial heterogeneity in the analysis of electroencephalogram data. It is shown that by transforming the electroencephalogram time series from the time into the frequency domain, one can describe the data by a generalized linear model. On the basis of this result a covariate-adjusted finite mixture model is developed to model spatial variability of electrical scalp activity.

Investigating and Analyzing Heterogeneity in Meta-analysis

Meta-analysis is increasingly being used to summarize the evidence provided by clinical trials and observational studies. Meta-analysis involves providing a report of primary research using statistical methods and analysis. Chapter 7 first reviews the statistical methods applied in meta-analysis and then introduces new contributions to the field.

The first involves the analysis of heterogeneity, which is a crucial part of each meta-analysis. To analyze heterogeneity, often a random effects model, which incorporates variation between studies, is considered. It is assumed that each study has its own (true) exposure or therapy effect and that there is a random distribution of these true exposure effects around a central effect. In other words, the random effects model allows nonhomogeneity between the effects of different studies. The variability between studies is quantified by the heterogeneity variance τ^2. To compare the performance of four estimators of τ^2, a simulation study was performed. This study compared the DerSimonian–Laird estimator described in Sect. 7.3.1 with the maximum likelihood estimator based on the normal distribution for the random effects described in Sect. 7.3.2. Further comparators were the simple heterogeneity variance estimator described in Sect. 7.3.3 and the finite mixture model approach described in Sect. 7.3.5. The simulation study investigated bias, standard deviation, and mean square error of all four estimators of τ^2. On the basis of this study it turned out that the simple heterogeneity estimator behaves well for almost all settings. Additionally it is easy to compute. One drawback is that it relies on the assumption of a normal distribution of the random effects. If one is in doubt regarding this assumption, a finite mixture model may be considered. This estimator had the second-best properties in terms of bias and mean square error; however, considering ease of implementation and performance, the simple heterogeneity estimator seems to be a good choice.

Then covariate-adjusted mixture models are introduced as a tool in metaregression. Here, heterogeneity between studies is explained by known covariates while allowing for residual heterogeneity. By including covariates in the finite mixture model, one combines two approaches to meta-analysis, i.e., the approach of identifying heterogeneity and the approach of explaining heterogeneity by the means of metaregression are combined. In contrast to the usual random effects metaregression, the assumption of a normal distribution of the random effects is no longer required. Hence, if that assumption is violated, covariate-adjusted mixture models provide a useful alternative to standard random effects metaregression.

The book also introduces a meta-analysis on Aspirin use and chemoprevention of breast cancer in women. Here, also a discussion of how to perform a dose-response analysis within a meta-analysis is introduced.

Analysis of Gene Expression Data

The analysis of gene expression data is a rapidly growing field of medical research with a large and rapidly increasing body of statistical literature on the analysis of microarray data. Chapter 8 deals with the analysis of differentially expressed genes, i.e., finding differences in gene expression levels between subgroups of individuals. First, approaches based on hypothesis tests are reviewed and the use of mixture models in this setting is demonstrated.

Another part of this chapter introduces the use of meta-analytic methods for the analysis of differential gene expression. This method is applied to a famous data set dealing with the identification of the gene signature useful for breast cancer prognosis.

Chapter 2
Introduction: Heterogeneity in Medicine

Patients are not alike. In a therapeutic setting patients react differently to treatment regimes. Some patients do not respond to the treatment at all and others recover quickly under the treatment. This may depend on known factors such as genetic polymorphisms. For example, drugs known as beta blockers, which antagonize the beta-adrenergic receptor, are an important component of the treatment regimen for chronic heart failure (CHF). Genetic heterogeneity at the level of the beta-adrenergic receptor is thought to be a factor explaining the variable responses of CHF patients to beta blockade (DeGeorge and Koch 2007). Subsequent trials in search of personalized treatment of heart failure can take this genetic heterogeneity into account.

However, often the underlying mechanism that causes variability of treatment effects is not known; thus, the modest benefit observed in many clinical trials can be misleading because moderate average effects may be a mixture of substantial benefits for some, little, or no benefit for many and harm for a few. This is a case of unobserved heterogeneity of patients or populations since it is not possible to directly observe to which subpopulation a patient belongs. Likewise in this case, the underlying covariate which causes the variability in treatment response is not known.

From a statistical point of view this warrants a method which identifies the presence of unobserved heterogeneity and in a second step enables us to take known covariates into account to explain some of the heterogeneity. This leads to subject-specific or random effects models. In this type of modeling one is interested in investigating the individual departures from the mean response in order to analyze the results at the level of the individual patient. In these models the variability between individuals is assumed to follow a random distribution. In principle this can be any proper distribution.

This work focuses on a discrete unobserved distribution for the variability between individuals, which leads to finite mixture models.

Coming back to the possible outcome of a clinical trial with a modest average effect, there are three latent subpopulations: one with substantial benefit, one with little benefit, and one subpopulation which is harmed. The idea of a finite mixture model is now to estimate the proportion of these respective subpopulations and the

P. Schlattmann, *Medical Applications of Finite Mixture Models*,
Statistics for Biology and Health, DOI: 10.1007/978-3-540-68651-4_2,
© Springer-Verlag Berlin Hiedelberg 2009

corresponding mean treatment effect in these groups. This approach resembles an analysis of variance, albeit the membership of an individual to a certain subpopulation is not known. As an example consider the outcome of a fictitious clinical trial dealing with asthma. Here improvement of the forced expiratory volume (FEV1) may be a dependent variable. Suppose that the average improvement of a new drug was 221 ml in comparison with a placebo. Let us assume that the population of these patients consists of subpopulations due to a genetic polymorphism which is not yet known. For simplicity we postulate that only heterozygote alleles and not homozygote alleles are of importance, which implies that only two subpopulations exist. In this mind experiment we assume that the majority of patients do not benefit greatly from the drug, that is 70% of the patients show an improvement of FEV1 of only 80 ml compared with the placebo. On the other hand, 30% of the patients benefit from an improvement of 550 ml.

In a first model we assume that the data follow a normal distribution, $N(\mu, \sigma^2)$, where $\mu = 221$ ml denotes the mean and $\sigma^2 = 40,000$ the variance. A second model takes the presumed heterogeneity of populations into account. It consists of a weighted sum of normal distributions with

$$y \sim 0.7 \times N(80, 22, 500) + 0.3 \times N(550, 22, 500), \tag{2.1}$$

where the common standard deviation is assumed to be 150 ml. These two models are depicted graphically in Fig. 2.1.

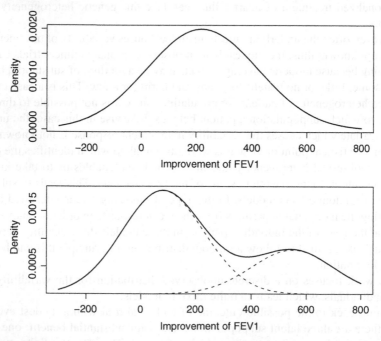

Fig. 2.1 Homogenous model with mean treatment effect $\mu = 221$ ml and a model with two subpopulations. Seventy percent of patients with little benefit ($\mu_1 = 80$ ml) and 30% of patients with considerable benefit ($\mu_2 = 550$ ml). *FEV1* forced expiratory volume

Table 2.1 Simulated data from a mixture of normal distributions

528.14	−49.63	283.65	152.99	472.42	365.29
672.86	167.65	649.12	338.38	612.13	115.80

Table 2.2 Simulated data from a two-component mixture of normal distributions with indicator variables z with regard to their component membership

Data y	z_1	z_2
528.14	0	1
−49.63	1	0
283.65	1	0
152.99	1	0
472.42	0	1
365.29	0	1
672.86	0	1
167.65	0	1
649.12	0	1
338.38	0	1
612.13	0	1
115.80	1	0

Table 2.1 shows simulated data from the second model. They correspond to the data directly observable by an investigator analyzing the results of the clinical trial. Mean and corresponding proportions of the respective subpopulations are not known. Likewise, for an individual observation it is not known to which subpopulation it belongs.

Now, if the component membership of an individual were known, estimation of the corresponding subpopulation's mean and the corresponding mixture proportion would be easy: To describe component membership, an indicator variable Z is introduced. If an observation belongs to the first component, the indicator variable z_1 will take the value 1 and 0 otherwise. For the second subpopulation the indicator variable z_2 is defined similarly. Table 2.2 shows the known indicator variables of the component membership of a certain individual.

Using the known indicator variables in Table 2.2, it turns out that the proportion of the first component equals the proportion of "ones" of the first component z_1, given by

$$\hat{p}_1 = \frac{4}{12} = 0.333. \qquad (2.2)$$

The proportion of the second component z_2 is simply

$$\hat{p}_2 = \frac{8}{12} = 0.667 \quad \text{or} \quad \hat{p}_2 = 1 - \hat{p}_1. \qquad (2.3)$$

In the same manner each subpopulation's mean can be computed. The mean μ_1 of the first component is given by

$$\hat{\mu}_1 = \frac{-49.63 + 283.65 + 152.99 + 115.80}{4} = 125.71. \qquad (2.4)$$

Similarly, the mean μ_2 of the second component can be computed as

$$\hat{\mu}_2 = \frac{528.14 + 472.42 + \cdots + 338.38 + 612.13}{8} = 475.75. \tag{2.5}$$

Unfortunately, in general, component membership is an unobservable variable. In this case, a frequently used algorithm for finite mixture models (see Sect. 4.4.3), proceeds as follows. First, determine the number of subpopulations k. Then, provide a first guess for the relative frequencies $p_1, \ldots, p_k$ of each component and the associated mean values $\mu_1, \ldots, \mu_k$. Applying Bayes's theorem (see (4.38) on page 75 for details) this information allows one to calculate e_{ij}, which denotes the probability that the ith observation belongs to the jth component.

By replacing the unknown indicator variables with the probabilities of component membership, one obtains new estimates of the mixing proportions p_j and population means μ_j. This procedure is repeated until a convergence criterion is met. This algorithm is known as the expectation maxmization. A formal derivation and description of algorithms for finite mixture models is developed in Chap. 4.

In contrast to Fig. 2.1, mixtures of normal densities with two components are not necessarily bimodal. This is shown in Fig. 2.2. The shape of mixture densities of

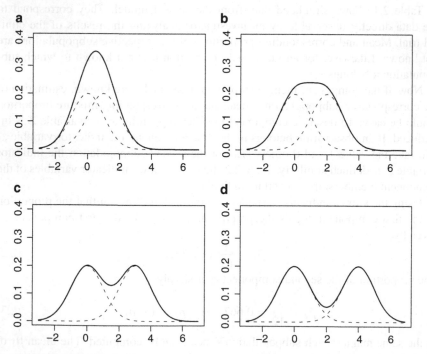

Fig. 2.2 Mixture densities with two univariate normal distributions with $p_1 = p_2 = 0.5$, $\mu_1 = 0$, and $\sigma^2 = 1$ in the cases **a** $\mu_2 = 1$, **b** $\mu_2 = 2$, **c** $\mu_2 = 3$, and **d** $\mu_2 = 4$

two univariate normal densities depends on how far the individual means of the two distributions are apart. Figure 2.2 shows mixtures with $\mu_1 = 0$, $p_1 = p_2 = 0.5$, and variance $\sigma_2 = 1$. If the difference $\Delta = |\mu_1 - \mu_2|$ is 1 (see Fig. 2.2a) the shape of the mixed distribution is unimodal. The same applies if the difference is 2. For $\Delta = 3$ and $\Delta = 4$ the resulting mixture distributions are bimodal.

Following this presentation of the general ideas of finite mixture models, Sect. 2.1 applies this model to data from an epidemiologic study.

2.1 Example: Plasma Concentration of Beta-Carotene

2.1.1 Identification of a Latent Structure

High intakes of fruits and vegetables, or high circulating levels of their biomarkers (carotenoids, vitamins C and E), have been associated with a relatively low incidence of cardiovascular disease, cataracts, and cancer. A high fruit and vegetable diet increases antioxidant concentrations in blood and body tissues, and potentially protects against oxidative damage to cells and tissues. This observation led to the initiation of randomized clinical trials focusing on subjects with a high risk of cancer. One of these trials is the beta-Carotene and Retinol Efficacy Trial (CARET) initiated by Goodman et al. (1993). This trial tested the effect of daily beta-carotene (30 mg) and retinyl palmitate (25,000 IU) intake on the incidence of lung cancer, other cancers, and death in 18,314 participants who were at high risk for lung cancer because of a history of smoking or asbestos exposure. CARET was stopped ahead of schedule in January 1996 because participants who were randomly assigned to receive the active intervention were found to have a 28% increase in incidence of lung cancer, a 17% increase in incidence of death, and a higher rate of cardiovascular disease mortality compared with participants in the placebo group (Goodman et al. 2004).

In a systematic review summarizing the evidence from controlled clinical trials Caraballoso et al. (2003) concluded that there is currently no evidence to support recommending vitamins such as alpha-tocopherol, beta-carotene, or retinol, alone or in combination, to prevent lung cancer. Likewise, the risk of development of nonmelanoma skin cancer was not found to be related to serum levels of any of the carotenoids measured in a study performed by Dorgan et al. (2004). Even worse, a recent meta-analysis of randomized trials (Bjelakovic et al. 2007) found increased mortality of patients supplemented with antioxidants.

Despite these disappointing results with regard to supplementation of antioxidants, the investigation of the determinants of plasma concentrations of micronutrients is still an ongoing area of research (Goodman et al. 1996; Margetts and Jackson 1996; Lagiou et al. 2003; Faure et al. 2006). A common finding in these studies is a negative association between cigarette smoking and plasma levels of beta-carotene. Many of the investigators mentioned before used a linear regression model to investigate the association between factors such as smoking, age, or gender and plasma

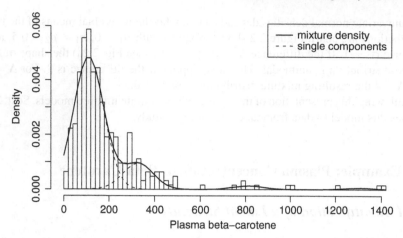

Fig. 2.3 Beta-Carotene plasma concentrations together with a four-component mixture model and single mixture components

levels of antioxidants. In our example, we use the data on beta-carotene plasma levels from Nierenberg et al. (1989) and Stukel (2008)[1] to address the following questions: Are there latent subgroups present in this data set and, if so, can this heterogeneity be explained by covariates such as age, gender, or smoking?

Figure 2.3 shows that there is wide variability in subjects. Especially the assumption of a normal distribution for these data seems not to be appropriate. For that reason Nierenberg et al. (1989) used a log transformation of the data to find determinants of plasma beta-carotene concentrations. But the multimodal shape of the histogram suggests that the data were sampled from a population which consists of several homogenous subpopulations.

Thus, the first step of an alternative analysis of these data tries to identify the latent structure. Using the methods described in Chap. 4, Sect. 4.4.5 leads to a solution which identifies four latent subpopulations. The first group has a mean concentration of beta-carotene of 126.05 ng ml^{-1} and constitutes 80.2% of the whole sample. The next latent population has a mean concentration of 350.83 ng ml^{-1} and forms another 16.8% of the total sample. The third subgroup has a mean concentration of 854.55 ng ml^{-1} and constitutes 2% of the population. Finally, the last subgroup has a mean concentration of 1,339.32 ng ml^{-1} and forms 1% of the overall population. The variance is assumed to be the same for each subpopulation and is 4,371.2. Hence, instead of a single normal distribution, these data can be described by a weighted sum of normal densities, that is,

$$f(x) = 0.802 \times N(126.05, 4371.2) + 0.168 \times N(350.83, 4371.2) + 0.02$$
$$\times N(854.55, 4371.2) + 0.01 \times N(1339.33, 4371.2). \tag{2.6}$$

---

[1] The use of the data for this book and the accompanying R package is kindly permitted by Therese Stukel, Dartmouth Hitchcock Medical Center, USA.

Looking at the fitted line in Fig. 2.3, we see that this finite mixture model provides an acceptable fit to the data.

2.1.2 Including Covariates

After identification of latent subpopulations, the question arises whether this latent structure can be explained by known covariates. The corresponding theory of covariate-adjusted finite mixture models may be found in Sect. 4.6.

In the simplest case this leads to a model with random intercepts. This implies that there are several regression models for each subpopulation which have the same slope but different intercepts. For example, consider the association of the amount of beta-carotene in the patient's diet with the beta-carotene plasma level of that individual. This covariate is labeled *diet*. In the Sect. 2.1.1 four subpopulations were identified. Now if the effect of diet is assumed to be the same in each subpopulation, this leads to the following four regression equations:

$$\hat{\mu}_{i1} = 109.80 + 0.0087 \times \text{diet}_i ,$$
$$\hat{\mu}_{i2} = 327.23 + 0.0087 \times \text{diet}_i ,$$
$$\hat{\mu}_{i3} = 812.30 + 0.0087 \times \text{diet}_i ,$$
$$\hat{\mu}_{i4} = 1303.52 + 0.0087 \times \text{diet}_i . \tag{2.7}$$

Since the effect of diet is assumed to be identical in each subpopulation, it is often called a fixed effect. This model is depicted on the left-hand side of Fig. 2.4. Here, the first component with the lowest intercept constitutes 81% of the total sample. The second component forms 16% of the population. As before, in the model without covariates the third component contributes 2% and the fourth component 1%. In terms of interpretation, the majority of patients have rather low beta-carotene plasma levels, 16% have intermediate concentrations, and only 3% have high concentrations.

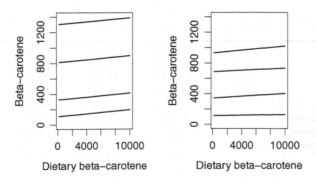

Fig. 2.4 Beta-Carotene data: finite mixture models adjusted for covariates. *Left*: A model with random intercepts. *Right*: A model with random slopes and intercepts

In a more complex model the effect of the covariate may differ in each subpopulation as well. This leads to a regression model with different intercept and slope for each subpopulation:

$$\hat{\mu}_{i1} = 113.56 + 0.0014 \times \text{diet}_i \,,$$
$$\hat{\mu}_{i2} = 342.69 + 0.0062 \times \text{diet}_i \,,$$
$$\hat{\mu}_{i3} = 687.04 + 0.0046 \times \text{diet}_i \,,$$
$$\hat{\mu}_{i4} = 930.32 + 0.0089 \times \text{diet}_i \,. \tag{2.8}$$

This is depicted on the right-hand side of Fig. 2.4. Now the effect of diet varies between subpopulations and is assumed to follow a random distribution; this is often called a random effect. The corresponding mixing proportions are given by $\hat{p}_1 = 0.8$, $\hat{p}_2 = 0.17$, $\hat{p}_2 = 0.02$, and $\hat{p}_4 = 0.01$. According to this model, 80% of the individuals have a small intercept of 113.56 with a small effect of dietary beta-carotene intake. Then there is an intermediate group with an intercept of 342.69 and a relatively large effect of dietary beta-carotene intake equal to 0.0062. Finally, there are two small subpopulations with large intercepts and a intermediate effect of the covariate dietary beta-carotene intake. After these preliminary considerations other covariates can be included into the model as well. Nierenberg et al. (1989) found a positive association between beta-carotene levels, dietary carotene, and female gender. Cigarette smoking and body mass index were negatively related to beta-carotene levels. Use of vitamins was also positively associated with beta-carotene plasma levels, whereas age was not associated with beta-carotene levels to a statistically significant extent.

Considering a covariate-adjusted finite mixture model, one obtains the results shown in Table 2.3. According to this model there are four subpopulations. The corresponding mixture proportions are given by $\hat{p}_1 = 0.8$, $\hat{p}_2 = 0.17$, $\hat{p}_2 = 0.02$, and $\hat{p}_4 = 0.01$. Again, the effect of dietary beta-carotene is different in these subpopulations. In the first subpopulation, constituting 80%, the effect is rather small, whereas

Table 2.3 Beta-Carotene data: finite mixture model adjusted for covariates gender, body mass index (*BMI*), smoking status (current smoker vs. never; former smoker vs. never), and dietary beta-carotene

Component	Weight $\hat{p}_j$	Estimate	Standard error	t	$\Pr(> |t|)$
Intercept 1	0.80	187.472	13.903	13.484	<0.001
Intercept 2	0.17	405.898	16.529	24.557	<0.001
Intercept 3	0.02	768.694	31.59	24.333	<0.001
Intercept 4	0.01	1,005.866	54.609	18.419	<0.001
BMI		−3.637	0.405	−8.980	<0.001
Current vs. never		−31.82	7.451	−4.271	<0.001
Former vs. never		−19.935	5.318	−3.749	<0.001
Female vs. male		32.950	7.105	4.638	<0.001
Diet 1		0.002	0.003	0.667	0.414
Diet 2		0.089	0.002	44.5	<0.001
Diet 3		0.042	0.009	4.667	<0.001
Diet 4		0.084	0.013	6.462	<0.001

in the fourth subpopulation the effect of dietary beta-carotene is much larger. Other covariates did not turn out to behave differently in these subpopulations. In accordance with Nierenberg et al. (1989) there is a negative association between the body mass index, smoking status, and male gender. On the basis of this model, vitamin use and age are not associated with beta-carotene levels to a statistically significant extent. In conclusion, this type of model has at least two advantages. First, we could identify subpopulations who react differently to dietary beta-carotene. This might be a starting point for further investigations. Especially of interest would be the question whether the recent adverse findings of supplementation of antioxidants apply to all patients similarly. Second, this type of modeling is one way to handle the problem that the data apparently do not follow a normal distribution. In contrast to, e.g., a logarithmic transformation of the data, the interpretation of the results remains on the original scale of the observations.

2.2 Computation

The previous models may be fit using the R package CAMAN. The first step in using the program is to load the package and the data set. This is done typing

```
> library(CAMAN)
> data(betaplasma)
```

The next step is to identify the latent structure of the data. To obtain a first impression of the potential number of subpopulations in our data the vertex exchange method (VEM) algorithm is applied. This algorithm is based on a fixed grid of potential means of subpopulations. The default in *mixalg.VEM* calculates the minimum and the maximum of the data and constructs a grid with $k = 50$ equidistant grid points. Then, the algorithm finds the corresponding population proportions that maximize the likelihood function. A detailed description of the algorithm may be found in Sect. 4.3.2.

The function is called with

```
> beta0<-mixalg.VEM(obs="betacaro",data=betaplasma,
startk=50,family="gaussian")
```

Here the call takes as arguments the dependent variable *betacaro*, which is the plasma level of beta-carotene. The number of grid points is set to $k = 50$. By default the mixing density is set to be the normal distribution. Also as a default the variance is set equal to the empirical variance. Typing *beta0* provides the following output:

```
> beta0

Computer Assisted Mixture Analysis (VEM):

Data consist of 315 observations (rows) four grid
points with positive support
```

```
    p              parameter
0.973285469   173.2653
0.017760636   895.2041
0.001319593   1299.4898
0.007634302   1328.3673

Log-Likelihood:   -2029.80100   BIC:   4629.10600
```

This result suggests that the data could be described by a mixture model with four components. In the next step we apply the function *mixcov*, which allows the inclusion of covariates into the model. The call is given by

```
> beta1<-mixcov(c(dep="betacaro"),fixed=c("1"),
random=c(""),data=betaplasma,k=4,family="gaussian")
```

This gives the (shortened) result

```
> beta1

Computer Assisted Mixture Analysis with covariates:

Data consist of 315 observations (rows).


mixing weights:
   comp. 1      comp. 2      comp. 3      comp. 4
     0.8026       0.168       0.0199       0.0095


Coefficients :
     Z1        Z2         Z3         Z4
  126.0613   350.826   854.549   1339.32978


Log-Likelihood: -1927.117      BIC: 3894.50
```

In the next step the covariate *betadiet* is included as a fixed effect into the model.

```
beta2<-mixcov(c(dep="betacaro"),fixed=c("betadiet"),
random=c(""),data=betaplasma,k=4,family="gaussian")
```

This results in the following output:

```
> beta2

mixing weights:
    comp. 1      comp. 2      comp. 3       comp. 4
0.811028183 0.157662064 0.021785704 0.009524049
```

```
Coefficients :
    Z1        Z2         Z3          Z4 betadiet
  109.855   327.232   812.343   1303.201     0.009
```

```
Log-Likelihood: -1924.664      BIC: 3895.349
```

Inclusion of the covariate leads to an improvement of the likelihood. Thus, not surprisingly, we deduce an association between dietary beta-carotene and plasma levels of beta-carotene. Next, we fit a model with the covariate *betadiet* as a random effect.

```
beta3<-mixcov(c(dep="betacaro"),fixed=c("1"),random=
c("betadiet"),data=betaplasma,k=4,family="gaussian")
```

This leads to the result

```
> beta3
```

```
mixing weights:
    comp. 1     comp. 2     comp. 3     comp. 4
0.80164319 0.16663101 0.01913382 0.01259198
```

```
Coefficients :
    Z1           Z2           Z3           Z4
   113.549      342.815      687.089      930.381

   Z1:betadiet Z2:betadiet Z3:betadiet Z4:betadiet
   0.001       0.006       0.046       0.090
```

```
Log-Likelihood: -1919.450      BIC: 3902.179
```

Comparing the log likelihoods of these models, we find again an improvement when we allow varying effects of the covariate in the respective subpopulations.

More covariates can be included into the model, for example, we might be interested in the effect of smoking status. Here, we use the treatment contrasts *current vs. never* and *former vs. never* The data set contains the variable *smokestat*, which is defined as a factor variable. By default R uses treatment contrasts for factor variables Now, the model is obtained with

```
beta4<-mixcov(c(dep="betacaro"),fixed=c("smokestat"),
random=c("betadiet"),data=betaplasma,k=4,
family="gaussian")
```

The result is given by

```
> beta4
```

```
mixing weights:
    comp. 1     comp. 2     comp. 3     comp. 4
0.81527849 0.15298759 0.01911870 0.01261522
```

```
Coefficients :
            Z1                    Z2          Z3          Z4
        125.882               354.613     704.594     959.963

smokestatFormer smokestatCurrent
        -20.667               -30.533

Z1:betadiet     Z2:betadiet     Z3:betadiet     Z4:betadiet
0.007           0.002           0.045           0.084

Log-Likelihood: -1915.798      BIC: 3906.379
```

2.3 Example: Analysis of Heterogeneity in Drug Development

2.3.1 Basic Pharmacokinetic Concepts

Pharmacokinetics investigates the absorption and disposition of drugs. Disposition is further subdivided into the investigation of distribution, metabolism, and excretion of a drug. Thus, pharmacokinetics is sometimes referred to as ADME (absorption, distribution, metabolism, excretion). A general introduction to the field of pharmacokinetics may be found in the books by Winter (2004), Rowland and Tozer (2005), and Tozer and Rowland (2006). The absorption characteristics of a drug depend on the properties of the chemical compound as well as on the route of administration and the exact formulation used. Obviously, this is not of interest for drugs which are administered by infusion or intravenous injection. On the other hand, absorption characteristics play an important role in the kinetics of orally administered drugs. The rate and the extent of absorption are important pharmacokinetic quantities for orally administered drugs.

Once in circulation, a drug is distributed throughout the body. Owing to differing characteristics of the various tissue types, this distribution is not uniform. Rather, areas of higher or lower concentration can be observed. Again, the chemical characteristics of the drug, and how it interacts with its surroundings at the molecular level, are determinants of this behavior.

Metabolism and excretion are the two ways in which a drug is removed from the body. Metabolism, which is also called "biotransformation," takes place mainly in the liver. The liver contains a host of enzymes, the cytochrome P450 (CYP) family, whose function is to dispose of chemicals that have entered the body (Pelkonen and Breimer 1994). These enzymes use iron to oxidize substances, often as part of the body's strategy to dispose of potentially harmful substances by making them more water-soluble. Bertz and Granneman (1997) found that 56% of 315 drugs were primarily cleared by CYP enzymes.

The products of biotransformation are called "metabolites." For some drugs, it is a metabolite rather than the parent compound that is the active substance. This applies, for example, to Dipyrone, an analgesic, antipyretic, and anti-inflammatory drug which is studied in Sect. 4.7.2.

2.3.2 Pharmacokinetic Parameters

The study of pharmacokinetics is a central part of drug development. For the analysis of pharmacokinetic data two different approaches are available. The first one is the so-called noncompartmental approach which relies on parameters such as maximum concentration C_{max}, the time of maximum concentration T_{max}, and the area under the time–concentration curve. The second approach is given by so-called compartment models. Compartment models describe the flow of a substance (chemicals, drugs, information) between the components of a larger system. In general, there are m components (the compartments) which may be linked to each other in any way. The flow rates or exchange constants between linked compartments are generally specified, and each compartment may also have output and input to and from the outside world. Compartments are described by differential equations. An overview of the use of compartment models in pharmacokinetics may be found in the books by Notari (1975) and Gibaldi and Perrier (1982). Basic pharmacokinetic parameters are defined and explained next.

Absorption Rate

In pharmacokinetics, absorption is the movement of a drug into the bloodstream. Absorption is often assumed to be a first-order process (Notari 1975), meaning that the rate of transfer is proportional to the amount to be transferred. In this case, the absorption rate (k_a) represents the constant of proportionality.

Elimination Rate

Similar to the absorption rate, the elimination rate (k_e) is used to refer to the proportionality constant in a first-order elimination process. Elimination refers to both biotransformation and excretion, and many processes can participate in the elimination of a drug. Here, k_e refers to the total elimination from all these processes. Elimination is usually well estimated by a first-order process. This implies that a constant fraction of the drug in the body is eliminated per unit time; thus, the rate of elimination is proportional to the amount of drug in the body. Even though some elimination processes may in fact be capacity-limited (e.g., in cases where enzymes are involved), the typically low concentrations associated with therapeutic doses imply that this usually does not affect first-order behavior (Gibaldi and Perrier 1982).

Apparent Volume of Distribution

The apparent volume of distribution (V) of a drug is defined by

$$V = \frac{x}{c},\tag{2.9}$$

where x is the amount of drug in the body and c denotes the concentration in blood or plasma. V is not a physical volume because the distribution of the drug in the body is nonuniform. It will not be lower than the blood or the plasma volume but for some drugs it can be much larger than the body volume. The volume of distribution is a mathematical factor relating the amount of drug in the body and the concentration of drug in the measured compartment, usually plasma.

Clearance

Clearance (Cl) can be interpreted as the volume from which all drug molecules are eliminated during a certain time span. This parameter is defined by

$$Cl = Vk_e.\tag{2.10}$$

Thus, clearance relates the volume of distribution and the elimination rate, and is a measure for the rate of elimination of a drug (Cawello 1999). The clearance is often considered to be the most important pharmacokinetic parameter (Gibaldi and Perrier 1982). Individual clearances can be defined for each elimination organ. Here only the total body clearance will be considered, i.e., the sum of all clearances.

2.3.3 First-Order Compartment Models

One of the simplest compartment models is a first-order oral compartment model. The principal idea is shown graphically in Fig. 2.5. This model can be obtained as a solution to a differential equation and describes the plasma concentration $c(t)$ at time t. The corresponding nonlinear regression model is given in (2.11):

$$c(t) = \frac{Dk_a k_e}{Cl(k_a - k_e)}(e^{-k_e t} - e^{-k_a t}).\tag{2.11}$$

In this equation k_a and k_e represent the constants of absorption and elimination, respectively, whereas Cl denotes the clearance and D denotes the dose given. This model implies that at the beginning the concentration–time curve is governed by the absorption constant k_a and later this curve is determined by the elimination constant k_e. This is shown schematically in Fig. 2.6. Equation (2.11) forms a nonlinear regression problem. In general there exist no closed-form solutions for nonlinear regression models. A solution has to be found by numerical techniques such as

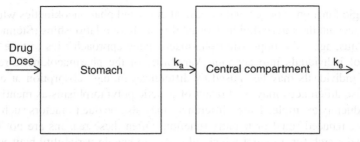

Fig. 2.5 The one-compartment model. The drug is absorbed from the gastrointestinal tract and then eliminated. k_a and k_e represent the rates of absorption and elimination, respectively

Fig. 2.6 Concentration–time curve based on an oral one-compartment model

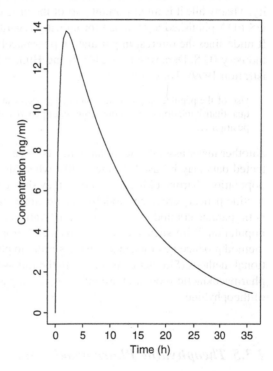

the Gauss–Newton algorithm. For details on nonlinear regression problems see the monograph by Bates and Watts (1988). Many of the algorithms proposed and described in that monograph are part of the R package *nlme* (Pinheiro and Bates 2000).

2.3.4 Population Pharmacokinetics

The foundations of population pharmacokinetic modeling were laid in the 1970s by Sheiner et al. (1972, 1977). This approach aims to model the relationship between physiologic function (normal and disease altered) and pharmacokinetics while taking into account the interindividual variability in these relationships (Steimer et al. 1994). Thus, again the population pharmacokinetic approach tries to take heterogeneity of individuals into account. Variability of the pharmacokinetic response between individuals may be caused by differences in, e.g., absorption or elimination. These differences may be a result of genetic polymorphisms as mentioned in the introductory example. These differences may also be due to factors such as age, gender, or reduced renal or hepatic function. Often these reasons are not known. Hence, we search for a model which allows us to handle variability between individuals due to unobserved covariates.

As a result, the population pharmacokinetic approach has been gaining popularity. Meanwhile it is an important part of the drug development process. In 1999, the US FDA published a guidance for industry regarding population pharmacokinetics. It underlines the interest in population pharmacokinetics within the pharmaceutical industry (U.S. Department of Health and Human Services: Food and Drug Administration 1999). They conclude:

> Use of the population pharmacokinetic approach can help increase understanding of the quantitative relationships among drug input patterns, patient characteristics, and drug disposition....

Another major asset of the method may be seen in the fact that sparse routinely collected data may be used. In the 1970s, when Sheiner et al. laid the foundations of population pharmacokinetic analyses, they showed that with data collected as part of routine patient care such modeling can estimate the average values of pharmacokinetic parameters and the interindividual variances of those parameters in a patient population. With such sparsely sampled data from patients receiving digoxin, their method produced estimates that were similar to published values derived with traditional methods (Sheiner et al. 1975). In the following section the ideas of population pharmacokinetic modeling are introduced using a data set on the pharmacokinetics of theophylline.

2.3.5 Theophylline Pharmacokinetics

Theophylline, also known as dimethylxanthine, is a drug used in therapy of respiratory diseases such as chronic obstructive pulmonary disease and asthma. Initial metabolism of theophylline is primarily performed by the hepatic CYP enzymes CYP1A2 and CYP2E1 (Tjia et al. 1996; Yoon et al. 2006). These data are taken from a phase I clinical study (Boeckmann et al. 1994). Figure 2.7 shows the concentration–time curve of 12 individuals whose theophylline concentrations were measured at 11 points in time after oral administration of one dose. Looking at these individual time–concentration curves, one sees a first-order oral compartment model seems appropriate. The individual dose given depends on the body weight of the subject.

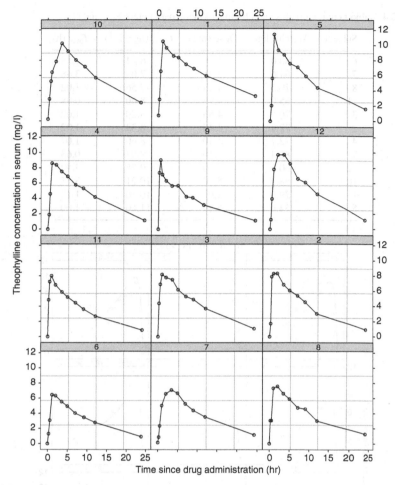

Fig. 2.7 Concentration–time curves of 12 subjects receiving an orally administered dose of theophylline

Table 2.4 shows the weight of the subjects, the dose given, and the noncompartmental pharmacokinetic parameters T_{max} and C_{max}.

The simplest possible pharmacokinetic model is given by a so-called pooled model which assumes for all individuals the same pharmacokinetic model with identical parameters for absorption rate, elimination rate, and clearance. The corresponding result is shown in Fig. 2.8. The concentration–time curves of these individuals differ since they have received different doses; however, the plots indicate substantial interindividual variability. It becomes clear that the assumption of homogeneity is too strong and that this model does not provide a satisfactory fit to the data. Since this data set consists of 11 concentration measurements for each of the 12 subjects, an individual model for each subject could be calculated alternatively.

Table 2.4 Subject characteristics and pharmacokinetic parameters T_{max} and C_{max}

Subject	Weight (kg)	Dose (mg)	C_{max} (ng ml^{-1})	T_{max} (h)
6	80.0	4.00	6.44	1.15
7	64.6	4.95	7.09	3.48
8	70.5	4.53	7.56	1.02
11	65.0	4.92	8.00	0.98
3	70.5	4.53	8.20	1.02
2	72.4	4.40	8.33	1.92
4	72.7	4.40	8.60	1.07
9	86.4	3.10	9.03	0.63
12	60.5	5.30	9.75	3.52
10	58.2	5.50	10.21	3.55
1	79.6	4.02	10.50	1.12
5	54.6	5.86	11.40	1.00

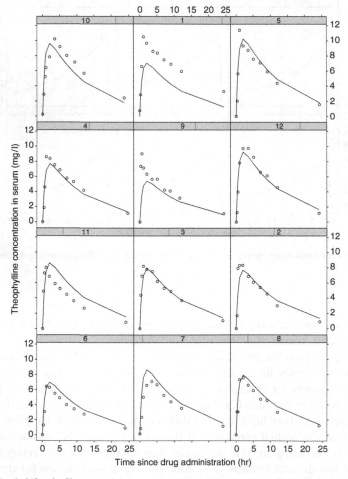

Fig. 2.8 Pooled fixed effects model for concentration–time curves of 12 subjects receiving an orally administered dose of theophylline

However, fitting a model to each individual implies fitting $12 \times 3 = 36$ parameters for the whole data set. As a result, this approach does not provide substantial data reduction. Thus, neither a pooled model nor individual models are particularly useful. One model for all individuals is too strict and one model for each individual does not provide sufficient data reduction. Additionally, many population pharmacokinetic studies do not provide sufficient data to be able to fit a model to each individual.

Thus, alternatively a random effects model can be fit to the data. Here again, variability between subjects can be modeled using a finite mixture model. In general, subpopulations with different absorption, elimination and clearance are considered. More precisely, there might be a subpopulation which has a large absorption constant but a low clearance. This would result in high, long-lasting serum levels of the drug. On the other hand, there might be a subpopulation with a small absorption constant but a high clearance. This would result in short-lasting, lower concentrations of the drug. For each of these subpopulations the elimination constant is assumed to be identical. In other words, absorption and clearance are assumed to vary between individuals and the elimination constant is assumed to be fixed. Technically speaking, absorption and clearance are assumed to follow a random distribution: They are random effects in the model.

The assumption of random effects for absorption and clearance but a fixed effect for elimination is motivated by Fig. 2.9. This figure shows the absorption rate, elimination rate, and clearance on a log scale for each individual together with a 95% confidence interval. It becomes clear that there is considerable variability between individuals for absorption and clearance, but less so for elimination. With these considerations a finite mixture model is fit to the data. The results are shown in Table 2.5. It turns out that there are three subpopulations. One subpopulation forms 34.58% of all individuals with a small absorption constant and relatively large clearance.

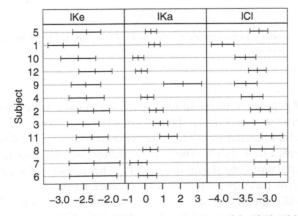

Fig. 2.9 Confidence intervals of individual one-compartment models of 12 subjects receiving an orally administered dose of theophylline, where lKe denotes the log of the elimination constant, lKa denotes the log of the absorption constant, and lCl denotes the log of the clearance

Table 2.5 Parameter estimates for the three-component mixture model fit to the theophylline data. Residual error is expressed as the standard deviation

Parameter	Group 1 (34.58%)	Group 2 (48.75%)	Group 3 (16.67%)
$\hat{k}_e$	0.082	0.082	0.082
$\hat{k}_a$	0.883	1.9332	2.409
$\hat{C}l$	0.038	0.042	0.028
Residual error		1.0247	

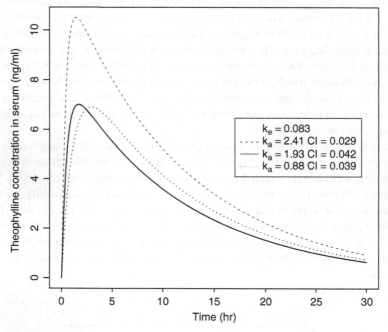

Fig. 2.10 Mixture model for concentration–time curves of 12 subjects receiving an orally administered dose of theophylline

The next subpopulation forms another 48.75% and has a larger absorption constant and higher clearance. Finally, the last subpopulation forms 16.7% of all individuals and is characterized by a large absorption constant $\hat{k}_a = 2.409$ and a small clearance estimated to be 0.028. The corresponding concentration–time curves of the three subpopulations are shown in Fig. 2.10. This model still needs to estimate a large number of parameters, that is, two mixture proportions, one elimination constant, three absorption constants, and three clearance parameters. Thus, a total of nine parameters were estimated for these data. To achieve more data reduction, a normal distribution for the random effects might be considered. In the simplest

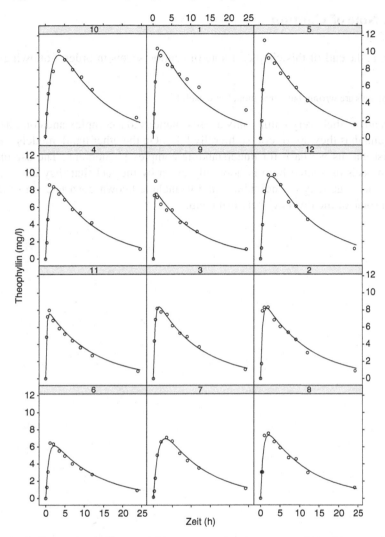

Fig. 2.11 Nonlinear mixed effects model for concentration time curves of 12 subjects receiving an orally administered dose of theophylline

case, e.g., only variability between individuals for the absorption constant would be assumed. This model has fewer parameters, but makes the additional assumption that the variability of the absorption constant between individuals may be described by a normal distribution. However, a satisfactory fit may be achieved if variability between individuals is assumed for the absorption constant and for the clearance. The corresponding estimated concentration–time curves are shown in Fig. 2.11. This model seems to provide an acceptable fit requiring only five parameters.

2.4 A Note of Caution

Finally, at the end of this chapter a note of caution seems in order. Following Box (1979):

All models are wrong, but some models are useful.

Models are by their very nature only approximations to a complex and complicated reality and thus they are of course literally false. On the other hand, models are the only instruments we have for understanding complex phenomena. The usefulness of the models presented here is hopefully given by the fact that they allow us to identify heterogeneity of individuals and to include known covariates in order to explain some of the diversity between them.

Chapter 3
Modeling Count Data

As already emphasized in Chap. 2, patients are not alike. Sometimes there is substantial variability between patients which cannot be immediately explained by known covariates. For example, the frequency of symptoms may show considerable heterogeneity. Often covariates which are responsible for this behavior are not known or not observable. As a result, this phenomenon is frequently called *unobserved* heterogeneity. From a biostatistical perspective the statistician needs to find a suitable model which identifies unobserved heterogeneity and which if covariates are available accounts for these known covariates. In this chapter this type of model is applied to count data.

3.1 Example: Morbidity in Northeast Thailand

In a cohort study in northeast Thailand the health status of 602 preschool children was checked every 2 weeks from June 1982 until September 1985 (Schelp et al. 1990). In this time period it was recorded how often the children showed symptoms of fever, cough, running nose, or these symptoms together. The frequencies of these illness spells are given in Table 3.1. The data set has been discussed by several authors (Böhning et al. 1992; Eilers 1995). Frequently for this kind of count data a Poisson distribution with $X \sim \text{Po}(\lambda)$,

$$\Pr(X = x) = \frac{e^{-\lambda}\lambda^x}{x!} = f(x,\lambda), \tag{3.1}$$

is assumed. On the basis of this assumption we obtain an estimate of the Poisson parameter $\hat{\lambda} = 4.485$. This simple Poisson distribution does not fit the empirical distribution of the data very well. Looking at the χ^2 goodness-of-fit test statistic, we find a poor fit ($\chi^2 = 3667.28$, 11 degrees of freedom with the last 12 cells combined).

A useful diagnostic tool for densities from the one-parameter exponential family are overdispersion tests which exploit the mean variance relationship of the Poisson

P. Schlattmann, *Medical Applications of Finite Mixture Models*,
Statistics for Biology and Health, DOI: 10.1007/978-3-540-68651-4_3,
© Springer-Verlag Berlin Hiedelberg 2009

Table 3.1 Distribution of the counting variable illness spells

Number of illness spells														
0	1	2	4	5	6	7	8	9	10	11	12	13	14	15
Frequency														
120	64	69	72	54	35	36	25	25	19	18	13	4	3	6

Number of illness spells							
16	17	18	19	20	21	23	24
Frequency							
6	5	1	3	1	2	1	2

distribution, which states $E(X) = \text{var}(X) = \lambda$. In the case of overdispersion the empirical variance of the data is larger than the variance explained by the model. A simple test for overdispersion exploits this phenomenon and was developed by Tiago de Oliveira (1965). This test has been referenced by Everitt and Hand (1981, p. 118) and by Titterington et al. (1985, p. 152). Böhning (1994) showed that the formula for the variance used for the test statistic was incorrect and developed the following simple test statistic:

$$O_{\mathrm{T}}^{\mathrm{new}} = \sqrt{(n-1)/2}\, \frac{S^2 - \bar{x}}{\bar{x}}, \tag{3.2}$$

which is approximately standard normal if the sample is from a homogeneous Poisson population with parameter λ. For the data at hand we have the statistics $n = 602$, $\bar{x} = 4.48$, and $S^2 = 20.44$, indicating strong overdispersion $S^2 - \bar{x} = 15.96$. This leads to the value of $O_{\mathrm{T}}^{\mathrm{new}} = 43.70$ and to the rejection of the null hypothesis of a homogeneous Poisson distribution. Assessment of overdispersion is still an active area of research. As an alternative to the test presented here, score tests may be applied. See, for example, the paper by Xiang and Lee (2005) and the application of the score test for overdispersed data in Sect. 5.5.2.

3.2 Parametric Mixture Models

The presence of overdispersion indicates that a simple Poisson distribution is not appropriate for the data at hand. As a result, a *mixture* distribution which takes this extra variability into account is assumed. Thus, if the Poisson parameter λ is not considered fixed, but assumed to follow a distribution itself, we obtain a mixture model. In the context of count data the negative binomial distribution described below can be thought of as a Poisson distribution with unobserved heterogeneity, which, in turn, can be conceptualized as a mixture of two probability distributions, namely, Poisson and gamma.

More formally, assume a family of densities $\{f(x, \lambda)\}$ parameterized by λ. Let Λ be the totality of values that can be taken by λ. If Λ is a (possibly infinite) interval and $g(\lambda)$ is a probability density function, then the marginal density $f(x)$ will be given by

$$f(x) = \int_{\Lambda} f(x|\lambda)g(\lambda)d\lambda. \tag{3.3}$$

One possible approach is to assume that λ follows a gamma distribution with

$$g(\lambda; \alpha, \nu) = \frac{\alpha^{\nu}}{\Gamma(\nu)} \lambda^{\nu-1} e^{-\alpha\lambda}, \quad \lambda, \alpha, \nu > 0, \tag{3.4}$$

where $\Gamma(u)$ denotes the gamma function

$$\Gamma(u) = \int_0^{\infty} t^{u-1} e^{-t} dt, \quad u > 0. \tag{3.5}$$

Then it follows that

$$\int_0^{\infty} f(x, \lambda)g(\lambda)d\lambda = \int_0^{\infty} \frac{e^{-\lambda}\lambda^x}{x!} \frac{\alpha^{\nu}}{\Gamma(\nu)} \lambda^{\nu-1} e^{-\alpha\lambda} d\lambda$$

$$= \frac{\alpha^{\nu}}{x!\Gamma(\nu)} \int_0^{\infty} \lambda^{\nu+x-1} e^{-(\alpha+1)\lambda} d\lambda$$

$$= \frac{\alpha^{\nu}}{x!\Gamma(\nu)} \frac{1}{(\alpha+1)^{\nu+x}} \int_0^{\infty} [(\alpha+1)\lambda]^{\nu+x-1} e^{-(\alpha+1)\lambda} d[(\alpha+1)\lambda],$$

with $z = (\alpha+1)\lambda$

$$= \frac{\alpha^{\nu}}{x!\Gamma(\nu)} \frac{1}{(\alpha+1)^{\nu+x}} \int_0^{\infty} z^{\nu+x-1} e^{-z} dz$$

$$= \left(\frac{\alpha}{1+\alpha}\right)^{\nu} \frac{\Gamma(\nu+x)}{x!\Gamma(\nu)} \left(\frac{1}{\alpha+1}\right)^x$$

$$\text{since } \int_0^{\infty} z^{\nu+x-1} e^{-z} dz = \Gamma(\nu+x)$$

$$= \binom{\nu+x-1}{x} \left(\frac{\alpha}{\alpha+1}\right)^{\nu} \left(\frac{1}{\alpha+1}\right)^x \tag{3.6}$$

$$= \binom{\nu+x-1}{x} p^{\nu}(1-p)^x. \tag{3.7}$$

This is the density function of a negative binomial distribution with parameters ν and $p = \frac{\alpha}{\alpha+1}$. Its expectation and variance are given by

$$\mu = \nu \frac{1-p}{p} = \frac{\nu}{\alpha} \tag{3.8}$$

and

$$\sigma^2 = v\frac{1-p}{p^2} = \mu\frac{1}{p}$$
$$= \frac{v}{\alpha} + \frac{v}{\alpha^2}, \tag{3.9}$$

respectively (Mood et al. 1974, Chap. 2). Johnson et al. (1992, Chap. 5) presented a series of methods for estimating the parameters of the negative binomial distribution. The method of moments simply equates the sample mean $\bar{x}$ and sample variance S^2 with the theoretical moments μ and σ^2. This leads to the moment estimates

$$\hat{\mu} = \bar{x},$$
$$\hat{v} = \frac{\bar{x}^2}{S^2 - \bar{x}},$$
$$\hat{p} = \frac{\bar{x}}{S^2}. \tag{3.10}$$

On the basis of (3.10), estimates $\hat{\mu} = 4.485$, $\hat{p} = 0.218$, and $\hat{v} = 1.237$ are obtained for the illness spell data. Estimation of the dispersion parameter of the negative binomial distribution is still an active area of research (see also Sect. 5.5.3 for a discussion of the topic). For a recent discussion of methods based on maximum likelihood see, for example, Saha and Paul (2005).

On the basis of these estimates the negative binomial density in Fig. 3.1 is obtained. Obviously, judging from this graph, this conjugate Poisson mixture model

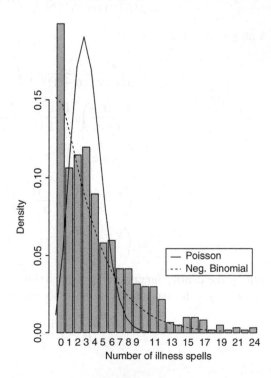

Fig. 3.1 Empirical density, Poisson density, and negative binomial density of the illness spell data

provides a much better fit to the data than a single Poisson density. However, the choice of the gamma distribution as the mixing distribution is somewhat arbitrary and is mainly guided by mathematical convenience. Likewise, looking at the χ^2 goodness-of-fit test statistic, we find a better, but still not a satisfactory fit ($\chi^2 = 36.217$, $p = 0.029$, 22 degrees of freedom with the last two cells combined).

3.3 Finite Mixture Models

Another potential class of models is finite mixture models, possibly adjusted for covariates. The books by Everitt and Hand (1981), McLachlan and Basford (1988), Böhning (1999a), McLachlan and Peel (2000), and more recently Frühwirth-Schnatter (2006) cover a wide range of applications of finite mixture models.

Frequently, we assume a one-parameter density $f(x|\lambda)$ for the phenomenon of interest. λ denotes the parameter of the population, whereas x is in the sample space X a subset of the real line. As already demonstrated for the illness spell data this simple model is too strict to describe real data. Thus, a natural extension of this simple model would be the *heterogeneous* case, where we assume that the population of interest consists of several subpopulations denoted by $\lambda_1, \lambda_2, \ldots, \lambda_k$. In contrast to the homogenous case, we have the same type of density for each subpopulation but different parameters λ_j in subpopulation j. In contrast to the mixture model, where a gamma distribution was assumed for the Poisson parameter λ, here no specific assumption of the form of the distribution of λ is made.

In the sample $x_1, x_2, \ldots, x_n$ it is not observed to which subpopulation the information belongs; therefore, this phenomenon is called *unobserved heterogeneity*. Now let a latent variable Z describe population membership. Then the joint density $f(x,z)$ may be written as

$$f(x,z) = f(x|z)f(z) = f(x|\lambda_z)p_z, \tag{3.11}$$

where $f(x|z)$ is the density conditional on membership in subpopulation z. Thus, the unconditional density $f(x)$ is given by the marginal density summing over the latent variable Z

$$f(x,P) = \sum_{j=1}^{k} f(x,\lambda_j)p_j. \tag{3.12}$$

In this case p_j is the probability of belonging to the jth subpopulation having parameter λ_j. As a result, the p_j are subject to the constraints $p_j \geq 0$ and $p_1 + \cdots + p_k = 1$. Thus, (3.12) denotes a semiparametric mixture distribution with *mixing kernel* $f(x,\lambda_j)$ and mixing distribution

$$P \equiv \begin{bmatrix} \lambda_1 \ldots \lambda_k \\ p_1 \ldots p_k \end{bmatrix} \tag{3.13}$$

in which weights $p_1, \ldots, p_k$ are given to parameters $\lambda_1, \ldots, \lambda_k$. Note that also the number of components k needs to be estimated.

Coming back to the example, we could use a finite mixture model of Poisson distributions instead of the parametric mixture model or the simple Poisson model

$$f(x,P) = \sum_{j=1}^{k} f(x,\lambda_j)p_j,$$

$$\text{where} \quad f(x,\lambda_j) = \exp(-\lambda_j)\lambda_j^x/x!.$$

This model assumes that there are k latent subgroups with parameters λ_j and corresponding mixing weights p_j. Thus, each subpopulation is described by a Poisson distribution with parameter λ_j.

3.3.1 Diagnostic Plots for Finite Mixture Models

An initial diagnostic plot indicative of mixture models is the plot of the logarithm of the *homogeneity* residuals obtained under the homogenous model against the observations. If a mixture is present, Lindsay and Roeder (1992) have shown that such a plot will be *convex*. A diagnostic technique which exploits the properties of the nonparametric maximum likelihood estimator (NPMLE) has been suggested by Lindsay and Roeder (1992). Details may be found in Sect. 4.3. The approach of Lindsay and Roeder focuses on the graphical analysis of the residuals

$$\frac{\text{Observed} - \text{expected}}{\text{expected}},$$

where "observed" is defined to be $w(x)$, the relative frequency of the sample elements equal to x. "Expected" is the expected frequency under the model considered; under the model $f(x,\lambda)$ we obtain the homogeneity residual $r_{\hat{\lambda}}(x) = \frac{w(x)}{f(x,\hat{\lambda})} - 1$, whereas $r_{\hat{P}}(x) = \frac{w(x)}{f(x,\hat{P})} - 1$ leads to the heterogeneity residuals. If the mixture models holds a certain pattern of homogeneity residuals plotted against the observations, x can be indicative of a mixture model. This is very similar to regression diagnostics where certain patterns are indicative of other models. Lindsay and Roeder (1992) have shown that a plot of $\log(r_{\hat{\lambda}}(x) + 1)$ should have a *convex* structure if a mixture model is present. The graph in Fig. 3.2 clearly shows a convex pattern and we conclude that a mixture model may be appropriate for the data. Again, a Poisson distribution is assumed for the mixing kernel $f(x;\lambda_j)$.

3.3.2 A Finite Mixture Model for the Illness Spell Data

For the construction of a finite mixture model it is necessary to make a choice with regard to the number of components k. Either we can treat k as fixed and known,

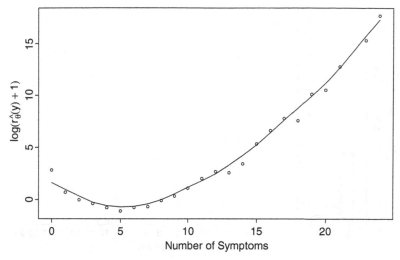

Fig. 3.2 Diagnostic plot of homogeneity residuals (*circles*) and the smoothed curve

which is called the *fixed support size* case, or the number of components k can be treated as unknown, which is the *flexible support size* case. In the latter case, we think of P as a completely unknown discrete distribution on the values of λ with at most n support points.

For an initial data analysis it is useful to treat the number of components k as unknown. This has the advantage that it may serve as a diagnostic for the number of components and that suitable starting values are provided for the algorithms for the fixed support size case model. This strategy is implemented in the program C.A.MAN (Computer Assisted Analysis of Mixtures; Böhning, Schlattmann, and Lindsay (1992), Böhning, Dietz, and Schlattmann (1998)). The functionality of the program is now available in the R package CAMAN, which is used for the calculations at hand. See also Sect. 3.4 for more information. In this program several algorithms for the estimation of the parameters of a mixture are available. These algorithms include the vertex exchange method for flexible support size and the expectation maxmization for fixed support size. A detailed description of the algorithms is given in Sect. 4.3.2. The description of the VEM algorithm is given in Algorithm 4.3.2 on page 69 and the EM algorithm is given in Algorithm 4.4.1 described on page 76.

The first choice in using the VEM algorithm for the flexible support size involves the selection of a grid of parameter values $\lambda_1, \ldots, \lambda_m$ over which we wish to find the corresponding population proportions that maximize the likelihood function. This forms the first step of a mixture algorithm. Here, using C.A.MAN, the NPMLE turns out to consist out of at least three distinct groups. A bar chart of the NPMLE is shown in Fig. 3.3. These grid points with positive support may be used as starting values for the EM algorithm. Combining coinciding parameter values leads to the following five-component solution:

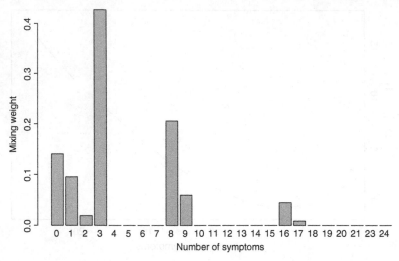

Fig. 3.3 Nonparametric estimation of heterogeneity for a sample of 602 preschool children in northeast Thailand

$$f(x, \hat{P}) = 0.0025 f(x, 0.0) + 0.1945 f(x, 0.1456) + 0.4799 f(x, 2.8175)$$
$$+ 0.2693 f(x, 8.1643) + 0.0538 f(x, 16.1559). \qquad (3.14)$$

This might be interpreted in such a way that there is a small proportion of children who are always healthy, another proportion who are almost always healthy, some who have intermediate risk of infection, some who have above intermediate risk of infection, and there is small proportion of children with high risk of infection.

3.3.3 Estimating the Number of Components

After having found the fully iterated maximum likelihood estimate, we might be interested in finding a parsimonious model. A natural approach would be to apply a forward or backward selection procedure to the data based on the values of the log likelihood for the respective model. Looking at the results in Table 3.2, we would conclude that a solution with four components seems to be appropriate for the data. The change in the likelihood from five to four components is negligible. As a result, the initial solution of the combination of the VEM and the EM algorithms overestimates the number of components k. A model with three components leads to a drastic decrease of the log likelihood. As a result, the final model is the model based on four components.

Table 3.2 Results of finite mixture model fit to the illness spell data

Components k	Parameter $\hat{\lambda}_j$	Weights $\hat{p}_j$	$\log L$	BIC
1	4.485	1	−2,135.422	4,277.244
2	1.823	0.646	−1,633.529	3,286.260
	9.236	0.354		
3	0.342	0.260	−1,573.427	3,178.855
	3.674	0.525		
	11.246	0.215		
4	0.142	0.197	−1,553.694	3,152.19
	2.812	0.480		
	8.145	0.270		
	16.140	0.053		
5	See (3.14)		−1,553.693	3,165.225

BIC Bayesian information criterion

Model Selection Based on the Likelihood Ratio Test

In order to apply a more formal procedure for the selection of the number of components k a generalized likelihood ratio test can be used. Statistical inference using the likelihood ratio statistic (LRS) for the number of components in a mixture model is complicated if the true number of components is less than that of the proposed model since this represents a nonregular problem: the true parameter is on the boundary of the parameter space. As a result, the limiting distribution of the LRS does not follow the usual χ^2 distribution. This is a well-known problem and still an area of active research. Lo et al. (2001) have studied the distribution of the LRS for various settings. One approach that has been found to simplify the asymptotic results while preserving the power of the test is to modify the likelihood function by incorporating a penalty term to avoid boundary problems. See, for example, Chen et al. (2001, 2004).

As a general result, the limiting distribution of the LRS has to be found by simulation techniques. One way to solve this problem for an individual data set is the application of the *parametric* bootstrap approach (McLachlan and Basford 1988; Feng and McCulloch 1996). This implies simulating from a certain mixture model under H_0 with $k = k_0$ and then fitting a model with k and $k+1$ components for these simulated data and evaluating the corresponding LRS. This procedure is repeated independently a number of times B and the replicated values of $-2\log\xi$, $\xi = \log L_0 - \log L_1$, $i = 1,\ldots,B$ formed from the successive bootstrap samples provide an assessment of the bootstrap, and hence of the true null distribution of the LRS. A detailed description of this approach is given in Sect. 4.5.2. This procedure then leads to a forward elimination procedure for the number of components k (Schlattmann and Böhning 1993; Karlis and Xekalaki 1999). Of course this procedure can also be used to perform a backward selection for the number of components of the mixture model.

Looking for a parsimonious model, we compute a model with a four-component solution and compare this with a model with five components. Computing the LRS, we obtain a value of 0.001 which indicates a negligible decrease in the log likelihood. Testing a three-component model against the four-component model, we obtain a value of $-2\log \xi = 39.466$. Thus, for these data a four-component model seems to be appropriate on the basis of the use of the LRS.

The Nonparametric Bootstrap Approach To Estimate the Number of Components

As an alternative procedure for the estimation of the number of components Schlattmann and Böhning (1997) proposed using the nonparametric bootstrap (Efron 1979, 1982; Efron and Tibshirani 1993). This approach is based on sampling with replacement from the original data and applying the mixture algorithm B times independently to the bootstrap samples. This gives an estimate of the number of components k for each bootstrap replication and hence we obtain the distribution of the number of components k. The mode of this distribution can then be used as an estimate of the actual number of components k. A detailed description of this procedure may be found in Sect. 4.5.3 starting on page 84. By simulation studies Schlattmann (2003, 2005) has shown that this estimator is mode-consistent in the homogeneous as well as in the heterogenous case when mixtures of Poisson densities are considered.

As a result, on the basis of the data in Table 3.3 we would conclude that four components are needed, which is consistent with the result obtained using the likelihood ratio test.

Looking at Fig. 3.4, we clearly conclude that this mixture density provides a satisfactory fit to the data. Looking at the χ^2 goodness-of-fit test statistic, we find a satisfactory fit ($\chi^2 = 3.444$, $p = 0.999$, 22 degrees of freedom with the last two cells combined). Summarizing, comparing the simple Poisson, the negative binomial (Poisson–gamma mixture) model, and the semiparametric mixture model, the finite mixture model with four components gives a superior fit. For a detailed discussion of when to use the negative binomial or the Poisson mixture model, see Joe and Zhu (2005).

Table 3.3 Nonparametric bootstrap distribution of $\hat{k}$ for illness spell data based on $B = 2,500$ replications

$\hat{k}$	3	4	5	6	7	8
Relative frequency	0.0004	0.564	0.3708	0.054	0.0092	0.0016

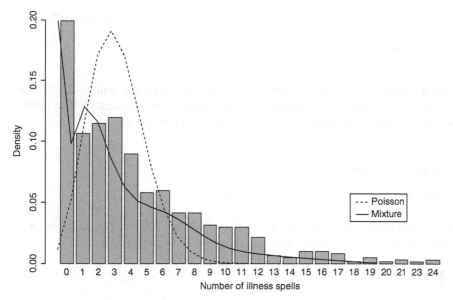

Density

Number of illness spells

--- Poisson
— Mixture

Fig. 3.4 Empirical density, Poisson density, and mixture density of the illness spell data

3.4 Computation

3.4.1 Combination of VEM and EM Algorithms

This section shows how to use the R library CAMAN to produce the result of the previous sections. The workhorse of the library is the adaptation of the program C.A.MAN written in Fortran and C by Böhning and Schlattmann to R. The library is named "CAMAN" and must be called with

```
> library(CAMAN)
```

The next step involves loading the example data from the cohort study in northeast Thailand. This is done using the command

```
> data(thai_cohort)
```

The function *mixalg* combines as a default the VEM algorithm and the EM algorithm. The first choice in using the VEM algorithm for the flexible support size involves the selection of a grid of parameter values $\lambda_1, \ldots, \lambda_k$ over which we wish to find the corresponding population proportions that maximize the likelihood function. The default in *mixalg* calculates the minimum and the maximum of the data and constructs a grid with $k = 25$ equidistant grid points. In this case this produces a grid of integers with $0, 1, \ldots, 24$ and the call of the function *mixalg* gives

```
> mix0 <- mixalg(obs="counts", weights="frequency",
  family="poisson",
> data=thai_cohort, numiter=18000,
  acc=0.00001,startk=25)
```

Here we assume a Poisson distribution for the mixing kernel, and each observation given in "counts" has frequency weights defined in "frequency." The option "startk = 25" determines the number of grid points. Then, typing

```
> mix0
```

gives the basic result

```
Computer Assisted Mixture Analysis:

Data consist of 602 observations. The Mixture Analysis
identified five components of a poisson distribution:

DETAILS:
             p      lambda
1 0.007138942  0.000000
2 0.189933532  0.149804
3 0.479856504  2.817818
4 0.269237565  8.164432
5 0.053833458 16.155972
```

This is the result of the combination of the VEM and the EM algorithms. A more detailed output is obtained by typing the command

```
> summary(mix0)
```

This gives

```
Summary of a Computer Assisted Mixture Analysis:

Data consist of 602 observations The Mixture Analysis
identified five components of a poisson distribution:

DETAILS:
             p      lambda
1 0.007138942  0.000000
2 0.189933532  0.149804
3 0.479856504  2.817818
4 0.269237565  8.164432
5 0.053833458 16.155972


number of iterations done: 8440
Log-Likelihood: -1553.811
```

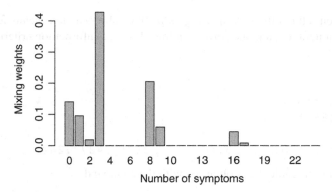

Fig. 3.5 Result of the vertex exchange method algorithm for a sample of 602 preschool children in northeast Thailand

```
BIC: 3165.225
accuracy at final iteration: 9.691139e-06

User-defined parameters:
 max number of iterations: 18000
 limit for combining components: 0.1
 number of grid points: 25
```

Useful information is given by the final result of the VEM algorithm. This can be obtained using the command

```
> vem<-mix0@VEM_result
```

This command returns a matrix with two columns. The first column contains the mixing weights p_j and the second column contains the grid points λ_j on which the mixing weights were searched. A plot of the grid points together with the mixing weights as shown in Fig. 3.5 may be constructed using the standard R function *barplot*.

```
>   barplot(vem[,1],names=vem[,2],
      xlab="Number of symptoms",ylab="Weights")
```

3.4.2 Using the EM Algorithm

Of course the EM algorithm may be used as a standalone algorithm. If the algorithm is used in this way the only thing the user has to do is to provide starting values. In order to construct Table 3.2 we could start with a homogeneous mixture model. This is done by typing

```
>   em0<-mixalg.EM(mix0,p=c(1),t=c(1))
```

This function returns the mixing weights p_j, the subpopulation means λ_j, the log likelihood at iteration, and the corresponding Bayesian information criterion (BIC).

```
> em0

  p   lambda
1 1 4.448505


Log-Likelihood: -2135.422      BIC:  4277.244
```

The next entry in Table 3.2 is obtained with the command

```
> em1<-mixalg.EM(mix0,p=c(0.7,0.3),t=c(2,9))
```

The starting values for the mixing weights p and the subpopulation means λ_j are expected to be given as vectors using standard R syntax. This leads to the following result:

```
  p    lambda
1 0.6457857 1.822729
2 0.3542143 9.235688

Log-Likelihood: -1633.529      BIC: 3286.259
```

3.4.3 Estimating the Number of Components

Apparently the log likelihood of the two-component mixture model is much better than that of the homogenous model. More formally, these models can be compared using the function *anova*. To apply the parametric bootstrap outlined previously in the section "Model Selection Based on the Likelihood Ratio Test," the function *anova(.)* can be used. This function takes as argument two objects of type *mixalg.EM*. The first argument is the model serving as H_0 with $k = k_0$ from which the parametric bootstrap observations are sampled. The second argument is the model presenting the alternative with $k = k + 1$. The third argument denotes the number of bootstrap replications B. For each bootstrap sample the LRS is computed and the percentiles of the bootstrap distribution of the LRS are returned.

```
> ll<-anova(em0,em1,nboot=2500)
```

This leads to the following result

```
> ll

   0.9      0.95      0.975     0.99
2.842339 4.551752 5.936260 7.793375
```

The observed value of the LRS is certainly much larger than any relevant percentile of the LRS distribution and the null hypothesis of a homogenous distribution is rejected.

3.5 Including Covariates

3.5.1 The Ames Test

Tumors arise and progress through the accumulation of serial genetic changes, including successive mutations, which involve activation of proto-oncogenes and inactivation of tumor suppressor genes, leading to the uncontrolled proliferation of progeny cells.

As a result, the identification of substances capable of inducing mutations is an important procedure in the safety assessment of drugs and chemicals. The Ames *Salmonella*/microsome test (Ames et al. 1975a,b) holds an eminent position among the tests available for investigation of a chemical's mutagenicity. Mutation can occur as a point (gene) mutation where only a single base is modified, or as large deletions or rearrangement of DNA, as chromosome breaks or changes or as gain or loss of whole chromosomes.

Mutagenicity is readily measured in bacteria when a substance causes a change in the growth requirements of the cell. The Ames test uses a number of *Salmonella* strains with a preexisting mutation which leaves the bacteria unable to synthesize the amino acid histidine and as result unable to grow and form colonies. New mutations can restore the gene's function and allow the cells to produce histidine. These newly mutated cells can grow in the absence of histidine and form colonies. The *Salmonella* strains used in the test have different mutations in different genes in the histidine operon. Each of these mutations is designed to respond to mutagenes with different mechanisms. Microbiological details may be found in the review by Mortelmans and Zeiger (2000). An overview of the historical development and the rationale of genotoxic testing is given in the review article by Zeiger (2004). To assess mutagenicity, several doses (usually at least five) of each test chemical and multiple strains of bacteria are used in each experiment. In addition, cultures are set up with and without added liver S9 enzymes at various concentrations. Therefore, a variety of culture conditions are employed to maximize the opportunity to detect a mutagenic chemical.

In analyzing the data, one takes the pattern and the strength of the mutant response into account in determining the mutagenicity of a chemical. All observed responses are verified in repeated tests. If no increase in mutant colonies is seen after testing several strains under several different culture conditions, the test chemical is considered to be nonmutagenic in the Ames test.

Table 3.4 Ames test: 4-nitro-*o*-phenylenediamine (4NoP)

Dose (µg/plate)				
0	0.3	1.0	3.0	10.0
11	39	88	222	562
13	39	90	233	587
14	42	92	251	595
14	43	92	251	604
15	44	102	253	623
15	45	104	255	666
15	46	104	259	689
15	50	106	275	692
16	50	109	276	701
17	50	113	283	702
17	51	117	284	703
18	52	117	294	706
18	52	119	299	710
19	52	119	301	714
20	55	120	306	733
21	61	120	312	739
22	62	121	315	763
23	63	122	323	782
25	67	130	337	786
27	70	133	340	789

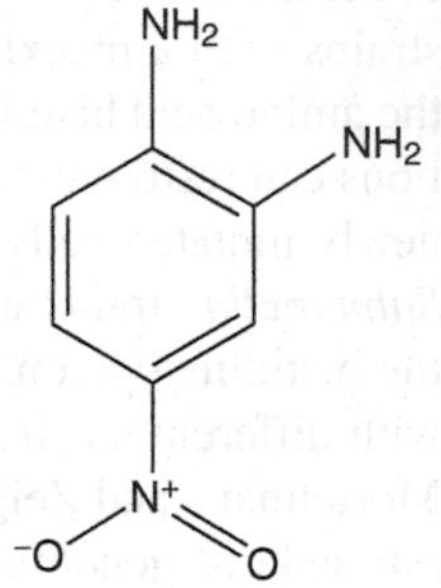

Fig. 3.6 Chemical structure of 4-nitro-*o*-phenylenediamine (4NoP)

Table 3.4 shows an example of Ames test data where a strain of *Salmonella* TA98 was activated with a homogenate of rat liver cells and exposed to 4-nitro-*o*-phenylenediamine (4NoP) with various doses.

4NoP is a nitrated aromatic amine (Fig. 3.6). This chemical is a component of both semipermanent and permanent hair dye formulations. The substance is frequently used as a comparator in mutagenicity tests. See, for example, Chung et al. (2000), Ajith et al. (2005), and Ajith and Soja (2006). The data in Table 3.4 were taken from Margolin et al. (1989) and denote the bacteria count for various doses of 4NoP. The primary question of interest is whether 4NoP acts mutagenically in the Ames test.

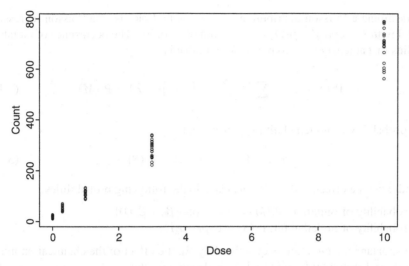

Fig. 3.7 Dose versus microbe counts of the 4NoP data

A plot of the data is shown in Fig. 3.7. Apparently the variance of the data increases with higher doses of 4NoP. This phenomenon should be covered by an analysis of the data.

In the analysis of the example data we employ a simple Poisson regression model, a model based on the negative binomial distribution (Lawless 1987), and a finite Poisson mixture model as suggested by Wang et al. (1996). The ideas and the notation of the respective models are developed in the following section.

Assessment of Mutagenicity

The primary issue in the analysis of an Ames test is whether there is evidence for mutagenicity. Unfortunately, the Ames test does not include a parallel assay for the toxicity of the test chemical. As a result, mutagenicity and toxicity have to be modeled and addressed simultaneously. Eckardt and Haynes (1977) proposed a model of mutagenesis and killing in the context of UV irradiation under the assumptions (1) the untreated cell population is homogenous, (2) the end points are measured all or none (mutant vs. nonmutant, survivor vs. nonsurvivor), and (3) stochastic independence of mutation and toxicity. Following these ideas, Margolin et al. (1981) proposed a class of models for the Ames test with the expected counts $\lambda(D)$ as a function of dose:

$$\lambda(D) = N_0 \mathrm{Pr}(D). \tag{3.15}$$

Here D denotes the dose in micrograms of the chemical, N_0 is the average number of microbes placed on the plate, and $\mathrm{Pr}(D)$ is the probability that a particular microbe will give rise to a revertant colony.

Assuming a Poisson distribution as given in (3.1) leads to a Poisson regression model with $\lambda = \exp(\beta + \beta_1 D)$ for the count of colonies. The occurrence of mutation implies that at least one colony is revertant, that is,

$$\Pr(X \geq 1) = \sum_{x \geq 1} \frac{e^{-\lambda} \lambda^x}{x!} = 1 - \exp(-\lambda) = \Pr(M). \tag{3.16}$$

The probability of no lethal hit $\Pr(S)$ is given by

$$\Pr(X = 0) = \exp(-\lambda) = \Pr(S). \tag{3.17}$$

Introducing the effect of dose D, this leads to the following probabilities:

- Probability of mutation: $\Pr(M) = 1 - \exp[-(\beta_0 + \beta_1 D)]$
- Probability of no lethal hit: $\Pr(S) = \exp(-\beta_2 D)$

Here spontaneous mutation is quantified by β_0, the effect of the chemical on mutagenicity is denoted by β_1, and toxicity is denoted by β_2.

Assuming (statistical) independence of the processes of mutagenicity and toxicity, the joint probability is given by

$$\Pr(D) = \Pr(M \cap S) = \underbrace{\{1 - \exp[-(\beta_0 + \beta_1 D)]\}}_{\Pr(M)} \times \underbrace{\exp(-\beta_2 D)}_{\Pr(S)}. \tag{3.18}$$

Here the term $\Pr(M) = 1 - \exp[-(\beta_0 + \beta_1 D)]$ remains to be dealt with. In the literature several proposals have been made. For an overview, see the review paper by Kim and Margolin (1999) and their Table 2 on page 115. Since $\Pr(M)$ is small, using only the first two terms of the Taylor series expansion

$$f(x) = \exp(x) = \sum_{k=0}^{\infty} \frac{x^k}{k!} \tag{3.19}$$

yields the approximation

$$\Pr(D) \approx (\beta_0 + \beta_1 D) \times \exp(-\beta_2 D). \tag{3.20}$$

In epidemiology, see, for example, Breslow and Day (1987), many observed dose-response relations for relative risks (RR) can be described by a power relationship of the form

$$RR(D) = (d_0 + D)^\beta.$$

This implies that the RR increases as a power function instead of an exponential relationship such as $RR(D) = \exp(\beta D)$. Breslow (1984) suggested this power model for the Ames test as well. The parameter d_0 is a nuisance parameter which either can be estimated from the data or in the simplest case is approximated in advance by the lowest positive dose used in the assay. This leads to the approximation of $\Pr(M)$:

$$\Pr(M) \approx \exp(\beta_0)(d_0 + D)^{\beta_1}. \tag{3.21}$$

Taking the natural logarithm of (3.15) and computing the expected number of counts and using the approximation (3.21) leads to

$$\log \lambda(D) = \log N_0 + \log \Pr(D)$$
$$= \beta_0^* + \beta_1 \log(d_0 + D) - \beta_2 D.$$

Note that the often unknown value of N_0 is incorporated into β_0^*. This model formulation has the advantage that the parameters of this log-linear model can be fit with standard software packages for generalized linear models (GLIMs) such as SAS or R.

3.5.2 Poisson and Negative Binomial Regression Models

From a statistical point of view the Ames test initiated a large body of research. An overview of statistical methods applied to Ames test data may be found in the review by Kim and Margolin (1999); see also Krewski et al. (1993). Besides the parametric and semiparametric models pursued here, also nonparametric (Wahrendorf et al. 1985) or test-based approaches (Bretz and Hothorn 2003; Hothorn and Bretz 2003) are available for the analysis of the Ames test. Early attempts to model data based on the Ames test used the assumption of a Poisson distribution for the count data. Margolin et al. (1981) demonstrated that this assumption is often invalid. They presented five sets of random samples of size 20, each under control conditions. They reported mean to variance ratios larger than 3.5 for two of these samples. They concluded that mixtures of Poissons should be used and applied the negative binomial model.

Poisson regression models belong to the class of GLIMs, which extend simple linear regression to distributions other than the normal distribution for the dependent variable (Dobson 2008). An overview of GLIMs is given in Sect. 4.6.1. The application of GLIMs requires the specification of an error distribution, which in this case is the Poisson distribution, the specification of a linear predictor which is given by a vector β of length $m \times 1$, and a design matrix X which has dimension $n \times m$. Together they form the linear predictor $\eta = X\beta$. Finally, a link function which maps the linear predictor to the scale of the error distribution is needed. In the present case we use a logarithmic link. Thus, the expected counts based on a Poisson model are given by

$$E(Y) = \lambda = N_0 \exp(X\beta). \tag{3.22}$$

For the data at hand this leads to the following Poisson regression model:

$$\log \lambda(D) = \beta_0^* + \beta_1 \log(d_0 + D) - \beta_2 D. \tag{3.23}$$

Here d_0 denotes a predefined constant, as before taken to be equal to the smallest dose. For the Poisson regression model we still have to deal with the variance mean relationship given by

$$E(Y) = \text{var}(Y) = \lambda. \tag{3.24}$$

Table 3.5 Poisson regression model: Ames test data with a strain of *Salmonella* TA98 exposed to 4NoP

Parameter	Estimate	Standard error	t	$\Pr(> |t|)$
Intercept	4.458	0.014	327.12	0.00
$\log(0.3 + \text{dose})$	1.163	0.023	53.84	0.00
Dose	−0.063	0.005	−12.44	0.00
Dispersion	0			

Frequently, this assumption is not valid and the possibility of overdispersion has to be addressed. Looking at Fig. 3.7, we see the variability of the data seems to be increasing with dose; thus, a proper model should take this into account.

This model, with results shown in Table 3.5, has a residual deviance of 305.28 on 97 degrees of freedom; thus, the ratio of residual deviance and degrees of freedom is 3.147. This indicates the presence of overdispersion. A problem associated with overdispersion is given by the fact that the standard errors of the parameter estimates are underestimated and need to be corrected. In terms of interpretation there is both mutagenicity and toxicity present. Toxicity is indicated by the significant effect of *dose* and mutagenicity is indicated by the significant effect of *log (0.3 + dose)*. For further comparison, note that the corresponding log likelihood for this model is −481.274.

Again, we consider the negative binomial distribution in order to deal with overdispersion. In the context of count regression models the negative binomial distribution can be thought of as a Poisson distribution with unobserved heterogeneity, which, in turn, can be conceptualized as a mixture of two probability distributions, namely, Poisson and gamma. For the negative binomial distribution the parameterization sometimes differs from that used in Sect. 3.2. According to (3.8) the expectation is given by $E(Y) = \frac{v}{\alpha} = \lambda$. As a result, $\alpha = \frac{v}{\lambda}$ and thus

$$p = \frac{\alpha}{\alpha + 1} = \frac{v}{\lambda + v}. \tag{3.25}$$

Thus, expectation and variance of the negative binomial distribution in this parameterization are given by

$$E(Y) = \lambda.$$
$$\text{var}(Y) = \lambda + \lambda^2/v = \lambda(1 + \lambda/v). \tag{3.26}$$

For the negative binomial regression model again a logarithmic link with $\lambda = \exp(X\beta)$ is used. This leads to the model

$$\log \lambda(D) = \beta_0^* + \beta_1 \log(d_0 + D) - \beta_2 D. \tag{3.27}$$

Owing to the extra parameter the negative binomial distribution is capable of dealing with overdispersion, as apparent in (3.26). Computation of this model may be done with the function *glm.nb* which is part of the R package MASS provided by Venables and Ripley (2002). Alternatively, software packages such as SAS and STATA may

Table 3.6 Negative binomial regression model: Ames test data with a strain of *Salmonella* TA98 exposed to 4NoP

Parameter	Estimate	Standard error	t	$\Pr(> |t|)$
Intercept	4.462	0.020	220.89	0.0
$\log(0.3 + \text{dose})$	1.186	0.032	38.01	0.0
Dose	−0.069	0.009	−7.66	0.0
Dispersion	108.695	36.232		

be used. Note that SAS and STATA use a different parameterization for the dispersion parameter v, namely, v^{-1}. The results of the model are shown in Table 3.6 and were obtained with SAS, Proc Genmod. The dispersion parameter v was corrected accordingly. The log likelihood for this model is -427.075, which is a much larger value than the log likelihood of the Poisson model (-481.274). The negative binomial model and the Poisson model are nested. However, the parameter v is on the boundary of the parameter space (e.g., the null distribution of the LRS is not the usual χ_1^2 distribution). Instead the asymptotic distribution of the LRS has probability mass of one half χ_0^2 and one half χ_1^2 distribution (Cameron and Trivedi 1998). As a result, to test the null hypothesis at the significance level α, the critical value of the χ^2 distribution corresponds to significance level 2α. Comparing the log likelihoods of the two models, we conclude that heterogeneity is present and that an additional dispersion parameter is needed. Here the dispersion parameter is estimated as 108.695. The residual deviance of this model is given by 106.285 on 97 degrees of freedom. The ratio of residual deviance and degrees of freedom is 1.096, which indicates a satisfactory fit of the model. The interpretation of the model in terms of mutagenicity and toxicity remains unchanged. Looking at Table 3.6, we see there is still a significant effect of *dose* indicating toxicity and mutagenicity is indicated by the significant effect of *log (11 + dose)*. However, allowing for variability between plates leads to larger standard errors for the regression coefficients. For example, the standard error of β_2 increases from $\text{se}(\beta_2) = 0.022$ to $\text{se}(\beta_2) = 0.031$.

3.5.3 Covariate-Adjusted Mixture Model for the Ames Test Data

Instead of a parametric mixture, a finite mixture model adjusted for covariates can be applied. We have the same semiparametric mixing distribution as in (3.13):

$$P \equiv \begin{bmatrix} \lambda_1 & \ldots & \lambda_k \\ p_1 & \ldots & p_k \end{bmatrix} \tag{3.28}$$

The major difference is now that the parameters $\lambda_1, \ldots, \lambda_k$ are no longer scalar quantities but vectors, e.g.,

$$\lambda_1 = (\beta_{01}, \beta_{11}, \ldots, \beta_{m1}), \tag{3.29}$$

where m denotes the number of covariates. In contrast to the homogenous case we have the same type of density f for each subpopulation but a different parameter vector λ_j in subpopulation j. The expectation of the ith observation in the jth sub-population is then given by

$$E(Y_{ij}) = \exp(\beta_{0j} + \beta_{1j}x_{i1} + \cdots + \beta_{mj}x_{im}). \qquad (3.30)$$

Estimation of the model's parameters is again performed by maximum likelihood, e.g., with the EM algorithm as outlined in Sect. 4.6. The results of the finite mixture model with covariates are shown in Table 3.7

The corresponding log likelihood of this model is -421.08, which is considerably better than the log likelihood of the homogenous Poisson regression model with a log likelihood of -481.27. The interpretation of this model is that there are three distinct groups in the data, which all have the same estimates for mutagenicity and toxicity but differ in their baseline characteristics. This is expressed by the three different intercepts. This result is in accordance with the well-known variability between plates of the Ames test. A graphical representation of the model can be seen in Fig. 3.8.

Table 3.7 Covariate adjusted mixture model: Ames test data with a strain of *Salmonella* TA98 exposed to 4NoP

Component	Weight $\hat{p}_j$	Estimate	Standard error	t	$Pr(>|t|)$
Intercept 1	0.298	4.319	0.025	174.358	0.0
Intercept 2	0.492	4.491	0.021	208.765	0.0
Intercept 3	0.210	4.581	0.026	178.055	0.0
log (0.3 + dose)		1.186	0.031	38.414	0.0
Dose		−0.069	0.007	−9.638	0.0
Heterogeneity	810.311				

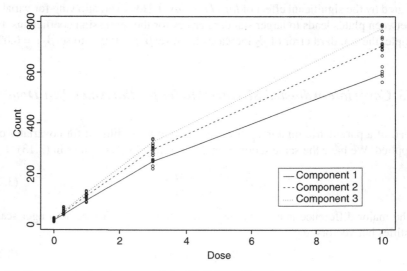

Fig. 3.8 Dose versus microbe counts of the 4NoP data with estimated regression lines based on a covariate-adjusted mixture model

Overall, there is considerable heterogeneity between plates indicated by the presence of overdispersion. In this example overdispersion was modeled using both a parametric and a semiparametric mixture model. Both types of models indicated that the substance is mutagenic and toxic (in the Ames test), while taking overdispersion or unobserved heterogeneity into account.

3.6 Computation

3.6.1 Fitting Poisson and Negative Binomial Regression Models with SAS

To fit these models with SAS the data need to put into the program. This may done by performing first a data step:

```
data nop;
input dose N; Do I=1 to N; Input count@@; output; end;
cards;
0 20
11 13 14 14 15 15 15 15 16 17 17 18 18 19 20 21 22 23 25 27
0.3 20
39 39 42 43 44 45 46 50 50 50 51 52 52 52 55 61 62 63 67 70
1.0  20
88 90 92 92 102 104 104 106 109 113 117 117 119 119 120 120
     121 122 130 133
3.0 20
222 233 251 251 253 255 259 275 276 283 284 294 299 301 306 312
     315 323 337 340
10.0 20
562 587 595 604 623 666 689 692 701 702 703 706 710 714 733 739
     763 782 786 789
proc sort; by Dose;
```

In the next step the covariate *logd*, namely, $\log(dose + 0.3)$, is computed:

```
data nop;
set nop;
logd=log(dose+0.3);
run;
```

With use of this data set a Poisson regression model is estimated using the code

```
proc genmod data = nop;
model count = dose logd /dist = poisson;
run;
```

The negative binomial regression model is fit with

```
proc genmod data = nop;
model count = dose logd /dist = negbin;
run;
```

3.6.2 Fitting Poisson and Negative Binomial Regression Models with R

The models presented before may be fit with R and the package CAMAN. We start with the Poisson regression model. The data presented in Table 3.4 are part of the package CAMAN. After the package has been called the data are loaded.

```
> library(CAMAN)
> data(NoP)
```

The calculations start with the construction of the variable *logd* given by $logd = \log(dose + 0.3)$, where 0.3 refers to the lowest nonzero dose. This variable is already part of the dataframe *NoP*. The homogenous model is obtained with

```
>  m0<-glm(count~dose+logd,family=poisson(),data=NoP)
```

This leads to the result

```
> summary(m0)

Call:
glm(formula = count ~ dose + logd, family = poisson(),
data = nop)

Deviance Residuals:
    Min          1Q      Median          3Q         Max
-5.09775    -1.17659    -0.02442     0.87859     3.61901

Coefficients:
            Estimate Std. Error z value Pr(>|z|)
(Intercept)  4.458168   0.013628  327.12   <2e-16
dose        -0.063136   0.005074  -12.44   <2e-16
logd         1.163001   0.021624   53.78   <2e-16
---

(Dispersion parameter for poisson family taken to be 1)

    Null deviance: 24783.24  on 99  degrees of freedom
Residual deviance:    305.28  on 97  degrees of freedom
AIC: 968.55

Number of Fisher Scoring iterations: 4
```

This model does not provide an acceptable fit and thus as an alternative a negative binomial regression model is fit to the data. Using the library MASS (Venables and Ripley 2002) allows application of the function *glm.nb*.

```
> library(MASS)
> m1<-glm.nb(count~dose+logd,data=NoP)
```

Typing *summary(m1)* gives

```
            Estimate Std. Error  z value  Pr(>|z|)
(Intercept)  4.462365   0.020187 221.054  < 2e-16 ***
dose        -0.069302   0.008563  -8.093 5.83e-16 ***
logd         1.186139   0.030746  38.579  < 2e-16 ***
--

(Dispersion parameter for Negative Binomial(108.1436)
    family taken to be 1)

Null deviance: 8515.51  on 99  degrees of freedom
Residual deviance:  106.29  on 97  degrees of freedom
AIC: 862.15

Number of Fisher Scoring iterations: 1

            Theta:   108.1
        Std. Err.:   27.6

 2 x log-likelihood:   -854.15
```

3.6.3 Fitting Finite Mixture Models with the Package CAMAN

The function *mixcov* of the R package CAMAN allows computation of covariate-adjusted finite mixture models. To fit the homogenous model the following call of the function *mixcov* is used

```
> m2<- mixcov(dep=c("count"),fixed=c("dose","logd"),random=c(""),
    data=NoP,k=1,family="poisson")
```

This call implies that *count* is the dependent variable, that *dose* und *logd* are independent variables, that *NoP* is the dataframe, that the number of components *k* is 1, and that the mixing kernel is the Poisson distribution. This gives the standard output

```
> m2

coefficients:
(Intercept)         dose         logd
   4.45817     -0.06314      1.16300

Degrees of Freedom: 99 Total (i.e., Null);
    97 Residual Null
Deviance: 24,780 Residual Deviance: 305.3    AIC: 968.5
```

To model the three-component covariate-adjusted mixture model displayed in Table 3.7 the following code can be used:

```
> m3<- mixcov(c("count"),c("dose", "logd"),c(""),NoP,
  3,fam="poisson")
```

This gives the result

```
> m3

Computer Assisted Mixture Analysis with covariates:

Data consists of 100 observations (rows).

mixing weights:
  comp. 1    comp. 2    comp. 3
0.2978747 0.4924652 0.2096601

 Coefficients :
    Z1      Z2      Z3    dose    logd
 4.319   4.491   4.584  -0.070   1.186

Log-Likelihood: -421.018      BIC: 874.2722
```

Chapter 4
Theory and Algorithms

4.1 The Likelihood of Finite Mixture Models

Estimation of the parameters of the mixing distribution P is predominantly done using maximum likelihood. Given a sample of

$$x_i \overset{\text{iid}}{\sim} f(x|P), \quad i = 1, \ldots, n, \tag{4.1}$$

we are interested in finding the maximum likelihood estimates (MLEs) of P, denoted as $\hat{P}$, that is

$$\hat{P} = \arg\max_{P} L(P),$$

$$L(P) = \prod_{i=1}^{n} \sum_{j=1}^{k} f(x_i, \lambda_j) p_j \tag{4.2}$$

or alternatively finding the estimates of P which maximize the log likelihood function

$$\ell(P) = \log L(P) = \sum_{i=1}^{n} \log \sum_{j=1}^{k} f(x_i, \lambda_j) p_j. \tag{4.3}$$

An estimate of $\hat{P}$ can be obtained as a solution to the likelihood equation

$$S(x, P) = \frac{\partial \ell(P)}{\partial P} = 0, \tag{4.4}$$

where $S(x, P)$ is the gradient vector of the log likelihood function, where differentiation is with respect to the parameter vector P. Maximum likelihood estimation of P is by no means trivial, since there are mostly no closed-form solutions available.

P. Schlattmann, *Medical Applications of Finite Mixture Models*, 55
Statistics for Biology and Health, DOI: 10.1007/978-3-540-68651-4_4,
© Springer-Verlag Berlin Hiedelberg 2009

Thus, a lot of research has been done to find reliable algorithms for the mixture problem at hand. Two cases must be distinguished:

1. The *flexible* support size case, where no assumption about the number of components k is made in advance. This case is discussed in Sect. 4.3.
2. The *fixed* support size case, where the number of components k is assumed to be known. Here the unknown parameters are the mixing weights p_j and the parameters λ_j of the subpopulation. This case is discussed in Sect. 4.4.

The algorithms used in the flexible support size case require some knowledge of convex geometry and optimization. Section 4.2 introduces the ideas of convex optimization in order to provide the necessary mathematical background.

4.2 Convex Geometry and Optimization

According to Rockafellar (1993):

> The great watershed in optimization isn't between linearity and nonlinearity but convexity and nonconvexity.

Many statistical procedures, such as least-squares estimation, are solutions of convex optimization problems. There exists a large body of literature on convex optimization. A comprehensive overview of convex optimization may be found in the book by Boyd and Vandenberghe (2004) which covers theory, algorithms, and practical examples. Another useful reference with regard to optimization from a statistical point of view is the book by Lange (2004). A more theoretical development is given in the books on convex analysis by Rockafellar (1996) and Hiriart-Urruty (2001).

In the following some basic definitions and important results of convex sets and functions are presented in order to provide the necessary background for the theory of semiparametric mixture models with flexible support size.

Definition 4.1. The set $X \subseteq \mathscr{X}$, with $\mathscr{X}$ a vector space, is convex if $\forall x_1, x_2 \in X$ and $\alpha \in [0, 1]$ the vector $x = \alpha x_1 + (1 - \alpha)x_2 \in X$.

Thus, in Fig. 4.1 the representation on the left is not a convex set, whereas on the right-hand side a convex set is displayed.

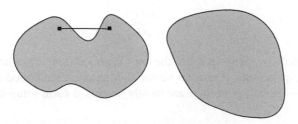

Fig. 4.1 Nonconvex (*left*) and convex (*right*) sets in the plane

A convex set has interior and extreme points. An interior point $x \in X$ can be generated by a linear combination of other vectors $\in X$ such as the point x_4. For an extreme point this is not possible. As a result, the points x_1, x_2, and x_3 in Fig. 4.2 are extreme points. More formally this leads to the definition of the *vertex* of a set

Definition 4.2. A point $x_1 \in X$ is a vertex of X if $\forall x_2 \in X$, with $x_1 \neq x_2$, and $\forall \alpha > 1$ the point $\alpha x_1 + (1 - \alpha) x_2 \notin X$.

Lemma 4.1. *Intersection of convex sets. Denote by $X, Y \subset \mathscr{X}$ two convex sets. Then $X \cap Y$ is also a convex set.*

Proof. If $X \cap Y \subset \mathscr{X}$, then for any $\alpha \in [0, 1]$ the point $x_\alpha := \alpha x + (1 - \alpha) y$ satisfies $x_\alpha \in X \wedge x_\alpha \in Y$; thus, $x_\alpha \in X \cap Y$ (Fig. 4.3). $\square$

Another important definition is that of a convex hull. For an arbitrary set X a convex hull is the smallest convex set containing X. It is denoted by $\mathrm{co}[X]$. In other words the convex hull of a set of points is the smallest convex set that includes the points. For a two-dimensional finite set the convex hull is a convex polygon.

Again, more formally:

Definition 4.3. Let X be a set in a vector space. Then the convex hull $\mathrm{co}[X]$ is defined as

$$\mathrm{co}[X] := \left\{ \tilde{x} \mid \tilde{x} = \sum_{i=1}^{n} \alpha_i x_i, \, x_i \in X, \, n \in \mathbb{N} \text{ and } \sum_{i=1}^{n} \alpha_i = 1 \right\}. \qquad (4.5)$$

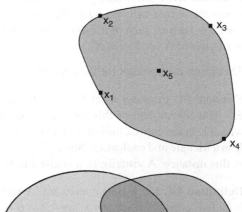

Fig. 4.2 Interior and extreme points of a convex set

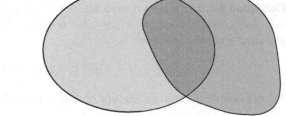

Fig. 4.3 Intersection of two convex sets

Fig. 4.4 Convex hull of a set

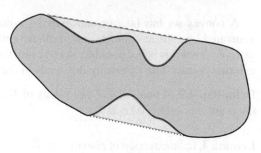

Fig. 4.5 An illustration of
Carathéodory's theorem for a
square in $\mathbb{R}^2$

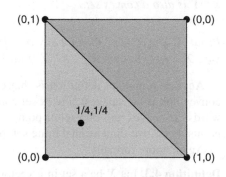

In other words the convex hull co[X] is the set of all convex combinations of elements of X. Figure 4.4 shows an example of a convex hull.

An important result from the geometry of convex sets for the theory of semiparametric mixture models is the Carathéodory's theorem:

Theorem 4.1. *Carathéodory's theorem on convex sets states that if a point x of $\mathbb{R}^d$ lies in the convex hull of a set X, then there is a subset X^* of X consisting of no more than $d+1$ points such that x lies in the convex hull of X^*. In other words, x lies in a d-simplex with vertices in X.*

This result is important for the number of components k of the mixture model.

Example 4.1. Consider a set $X = \{(0,0),(0,1),(1,0),(1,1)\}$ which is a subset of $\mathbb{R}^2$. The convex hull of this set is a square. Consider now a point $x = (1/4,1/4)$, which is in the convex hull of X. Then the convex hull $X^* = \{(0,0),(0,1),(1,0)\} \subset X$ is a triangle and encloses x. Since $|X^*| = 3$, it is easy to see that the theorem works in this instance. A visualization is given in Fig. 4.5.

Definition 4.4. Let X be a convex set. A real-valued function f defined on a set X is called "convex" if for any $x_1, x_2 \in X \wedge \alpha \in [0,1]$. If the inequality is strict, then f is a strictly convex function:

$$f(\alpha x_1 + (1-\alpha)x_2) \leq \alpha f(x_1) + (1-\alpha)f(x_2). \qquad (4.6)$$

As an example the convex function $e^x + x^2$ is plotted in Fig. 4.6.

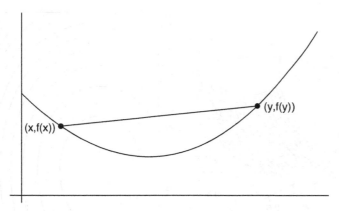

Fig. 4.6 The convex function $e^x + x^2$

Definition 4.5. Let X be a convex set. A function $f : X \to \mathbb{R}$ is said to be concave if for any points $x_1 \wedge x_2 \in X$

$$f(\alpha x_1 + (1 - \alpha)x_2) \geq \alpha f(x_1) + (1 - \alpha)f(x_2). \tag{4.7}$$

In other words, the function f is concave if the function $-f(x)$ is convex on X. Again, if the inequality is strict, then f is a strictly concave function.

Lemma 4.2. *Denote by $f : X \to \mathbb{R}$ a convex function on a convex set X. Then the set*

$$Y := \{x | x \in X \wedge f(x) \leq c\} \tag{4.8}$$

is convex $\forall c \in \mathbb{R}$.

Proof. We need to show the condition in Definition 4.1. For any $x, \tilde{x} \in Y$ the condition $f(x), f(\tilde{x}) \leq c$ is true. Moreover since f is convex, it follows that

$$f(\alpha x + (1 - \alpha)\tilde{x}) \leq \alpha f(x) + (1 - \alpha)f(\tilde{x}) \leq c \qquad \forall \alpha \in [0, 1]. \tag{4.9}$$

Thus, $\forall \alpha \in [0, 1]$ we have $[\alpha f(x) + (1 - \alpha)f(\tilde{x})] \in Y$, which proves the claim. This is depicted graphically in Fig. 4.7 for the function $f(x_1, x_2) = e^{x_1} + x_1^2 + e^{x_2} + x_2^2$. $\square$

Theorem 4.2. *If the convex function $f : x = (x_1, x_2) \to \mathbb{R}$ has a minimum on a convex set $X \subset \mathscr{X}$, then its arguments $x \in X$ for which the minimum is attained from a convex set. If f is strictly convex, then this set contains only one element.*

Proof. Denote by c the minimum of f on X. Then the set $X_m := \{x | x \in \mathscr{X} \wedge x \leq c\}$ according to Lemma 4.2 is clearly convex. In addition, owing to Lemma 4.1 $X_m \cap X$ is also convex, and $f(x) = c, \forall x \in X_m \cap X$. (otherwise c would not be the minimum). If f is strictly convex, then for any $x, y \in X$ and for any $x, y \in X_m \cap X$ for $x \neq y$ and $\alpha \in (0, 1)$

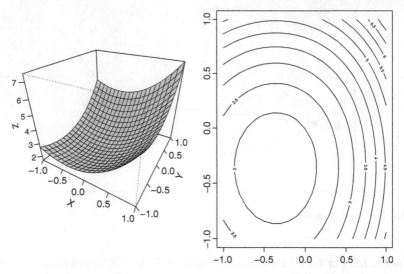

Fig. 4.7 *Left:* Convex function in two variables. *Right:* The corresponding convex level sets $\{x|f(x) \le c\}$ for different values of c

$$f(\alpha x + (1 - \alpha)y) < \alpha f(x) + (1 - \alpha)y = \alpha c + (1 - \alpha)c = c. \qquad (4.10)$$

This contradicts the assumption that $X_m \cap X$ contains more than one element. $\qquad \square$

Theorem 4.3. *Let X be a convex set with convex hull $co[X]$. Then for any convex function f on $co[X]$:*

$$\sup\{f(x)|x \in X\} = \sup\{f(x)|x \in co[X]\}. \qquad (4.11)$$

Proof. Let $\sup\{f(x)|x \in X\}$. As $X \subset co[X]$ $c \le \sup\{f(x)|x \in co[X]\}$. But on the other hand it follows from Lemma 4.2 that

$$Y := \{x|x \in co[X]|f(x) \le c\} \subset co[X]$$

is convex. By definition of c, $X \subset Y$. Owing to the definition of $co[X]$ this implies that $Y \subset co[X]$. Hence, $f(x) \le c$, $\forall x \in co[X]$. Finally, it follows that $\sup\{f(x)|x \in co[X]\} \le c \le \sup\{f(x)|x \in co[X]\}$. $\qquad \square$

Theorem 4.3 has an important implication for the construction of algorithms since it can be used to restrict search operations over sets X by subsets $X^* \subset X$ if the convex hull of the latter generates X. In particular, it can be used so that the vertices of convex sets are sufficient to reconstruct the whole set.

Theorem 4.4. *A compact convex set is the convex hull of its vertices.*

The proof is rather technical and may be found in the monograph by Rockafellar (1996). For a finite number of points the convex hull is called a convex polyhedron

Fig. 4.8 Convex polyhedron

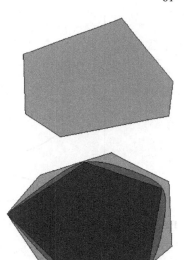

Fig. 4.9 Approximation of a convex set by convex polyhedrons

as shown in Fig. 4.8 and the extreme points of a convex polyhedron are again called *vertices*.

A closed convex set X can be approximated by closed convex polyhedrons with arbitrary precision:

$$\text{co}[x_1,\ldots,x_n] \supseteq X \supseteq \text{co}[y_1,\ldots,y_m]. \tag{4.12}$$

This is shown schematically in Fig. 4.9.

4.2.1 Derivatives and Directional Derivatives of Convex Functions

Proposition 4.1. *Let $f(x)$ be a continuously differentiable function on the open convex set $X \subset \mathbb{R}^d$ with gradient $\nabla f(x) = \left(\frac{\partial f(x)}{\partial x_1}, \frac{\partial f(x)}{\partial x_2}, \ldots, \frac{\partial f(x)}{\partial x_d}\right)$. Then $f(x)$ is convex if and only if*

$$f(y) \geq f(x) + \nabla f(x)^{\mathrm{T}}(y-x) \quad \forall x,y \in X. \tag{4.13}$$

Additionally $f(x)$ is strictly convex if and only if strict inequality holds in (4.13) $\forall y \neq x$.

Proof. We can arrange (4.6) to

$$f(\alpha x + (1-\alpha)y) \leq \alpha f(x) + (1-\alpha)f(y)$$
$$\Leftrightarrow f(\alpha x + (1-\alpha)y) \leq \alpha f(x) + f(x) - f(x) + (1-\alpha)f(y)$$
$$\Leftrightarrow \frac{f(\alpha x + (1-\alpha)y) - f(x)}{1-\alpha} \leq f(y) - f(x).$$

$\square$

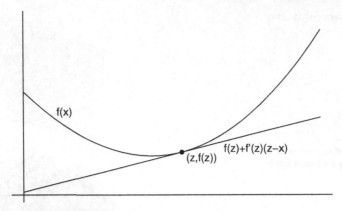

Fig. 4.10 The convex function $e^x + x^2$ with a tangent below the curve

For $\alpha \to 1$ inequality (4.13) is proven. To show the converse let $z = \alpha x + (1 - \alpha)y$. Then with some notational changes

$$f(x) \geq f(z) + \nabla f(z)^{\mathrm{T}}(x - z),$$
$$f(y) \geq f(z) + \nabla f(z)^{\mathrm{T}}(y - z).$$

Multiplying the first of these inequalities by α and the second by $1 - \alpha$ and adding the results leads to

$$\alpha f(x) + (1 - \alpha)f(y) \geq f(z) + \nabla f(z)(z - z) = f(z). \qquad (4.14)$$

This is just inequality (4.13). The proof for strict convexity is performed accordingly. Figure 4.10 illustrates how a tangent line to a convex curve lies below the curve. In other words the first-order approximation of f is the global underestimator.

It is certainly useful to have simpler tests for convexity than those of (4.6) and (4.13). This leads to the following proposition:

Proposition 4.2. *Let $f(x)$ be a twice continuously differentiable function $f(x)$ on the open convex set $X \subset \mathbb{R}^d$. If the Hessian $\nabla^2 f(x) = \frac{\partial^2 f(x)}{\partial x_i \partial x_j}$ is positive semidefinite, then $f(x)$ is convex. If $\nabla^2 f(x)$ is positive definite, then $f(x)$ is strictly convex.*

A proof of the proposition may be found in the book by Lange (2004, Chap. 5).

Example 4.2. The least-squares objective function minimize $f(\beta) = \|y - X\beta\|_2^2$ is convex. To see this consider

$$\nabla f(\beta) = 2X^{\mathrm{T}}(X\beta - y), \quad \nabla^2 f(\beta) = 2X^{\mathrm{T}}X \geq 0. \qquad (4.15)$$

Directional Derivative

The idea of a directional derivative is first developed using a one-dimensional function $f : \mathbb{R} \to \mathbb{R}$. If f is a convex function and $x < y < z$, then

$$\frac{f(y) - f(x)}{y - x} \leq \frac{f(z) - f(x)}{z - x} \leq \frac{f(z) - f(y)}{z - y}. \tag{4.16}$$

This is depicted in Fig. 4.11. Careful examination of the inequalities in (4.16) leads to the conclusion that the slope

$$\frac{f(y) - f(x)}{x - y}$$

is bounded below and increases in y for x fixed. Likewise, this slope is bounded above and increases in x for y fixed. On the basis of this result it is clear that left and right directional derivatives exist with

$$f^+(x) = \lim_{\alpha \to 0} \frac{f(x + \alpha) - f(x)}{\alpha}, \tag{4.17}$$

$$f^-(x) = \lim_{\alpha \to 0} \frac{f(x) - f(x - \alpha)}{\alpha}. \tag{4.18}$$

The concept of directional derivatives can be generalized to multiple dimensions. If $f : \mathbb{R}^d \to \mathbb{R}$, then the directional derivative of f at x in the direction $y \neq 0$ is defined as

$$\Phi(x, y) = \lim_{\alpha \to 0} \frac{f(x + \alpha y) - f(x)}{\alpha}. \tag{4.19}$$

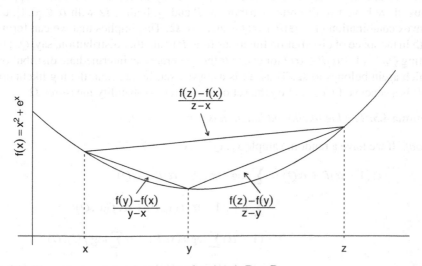

Fig. 4.11 Three-slopes relation for a convex function $f : \mathbb{R} \to \mathbb{R}$

Note that the directional derivative can be expressed as the inner product of the gradient $\nabla f(x)$ and y. If f is continuously differentiable, then $\Phi(x,y) = \nabla f(x)^T y$.

4.3 Application to the Flexible Support Size Case

Algorithms with flexible support size, i.e., when the number of mixture components k is not fixed in advance, are based on results of the topology and geometry of the likelihood.

Looking at algorithms for the flexible support size case leads to the mixture nonparametric maximum likelihood estimator (NPMLE) theorem (Böhning 1982; Lindsay 1983a,b, 1995). The idea of finding a NPMLE of a latent distribution has a long tradition. Substantial theoretical development was provided by Kiefer and Wolfowitz (1956), but there has been no development of numerical methods to use these results. The development of such methods together with further properties of the estimator $\hat{P}$ arose in papers that were published 20 and more years later. Particularly, Simar (1976), Laird (1978), Jewell (1982), Böhning (1982), and Lindsay (1983a,b, 1995) made major contributions to the field. In the following the most important developments will be summarized.

4.3.1 Geometric Characterization

One of the key tools to understand the nature of the NPMLE is to characterize the maximization problem in geometric terms. In the *flexible support size* case, i.e., with k not fixed, P may vary in the set of all probability measures with finite support. Thus, if we have two discrete distributions P and Q, both $\in \Omega$ with $\alpha \in [0,1]$, the convex combination $(1-\alpha)P + \alpha Q$ is again in Ω. This implies that we can form a path in the space of distribution functions from P to another distribution, say, Q_α; by letting $Q_\alpha = (1-\alpha)P + \alpha Q$ for every α this generates an intermediate distribution, which again belongs to Ω. Thus, Ω is a convex set. In addition, the log likelihood $l(P)$ is a concave functional on the set of all discrete probability measures Ω.

Lemma 4.3. *The log likelihood function is concave on* Ω.

Proof. If we have a random sample $x_1, x_2, \ldots, x_n$

$$
\begin{aligned}
\ell((1-\alpha)P + \alpha Q) &= \sum_i \log f(x_i, (1-\alpha)P + \alpha Q) \\
&= \sum_i \log \left[(1-\alpha)f(x_i, P) + \alpha(f(x_i, Q)) \right] \\
&> (1-\alpha)\sum_i \log f(x_i, P) + \alpha \sum_i \log f(x_i, Q) \\
&= (1-\alpha)\ell(P) + \alpha\ell(Q).
\end{aligned}
$$

The proof only uses the fact that the logarithm is a concave function that is
$\log[(1-\alpha)x+\alpha y] \geq (1-\alpha)\log x + \alpha \log y$. $\square$

These two results form the basis for the strong results of nonparametric mixture distributions. In particular, owing to Theorem 4.2 we know that a global maximum exists.

Now the task to deal with is to find the mixing distribution P that maximizes the likelihood

$$L(P) = \prod_{i=1}^{n} L_i(P) = \prod_{i=1}^{n} L_i, \quad \text{with} \quad L_i = \sum_{j=1}^{k} p_j f(x_i, \lambda_j) \qquad (4.20)$$

over the set of all distributions Ω. If we have a random sample $x_1, x_2, \ldots, x_n$, the objective function takes the form

$$\ell(P) = \sum_{i=1}^{n} \log \sum_{j=1}^{k} p_j f(x_i, \lambda_j). \qquad (4.21)$$

The problem of finding $\hat{P}$ that maximizes $\ell(P)$ over all possibly infinitely many distributions $P \in \Omega$ is obviously hard to solve. If the data are discrete, for example, categorical, then many of the x_i will be the same and there will be m distinct observations. Thus, each of the $x_i, i = 1, \ldots, m$ will occur w_i times. Now the log likelihood takes the form

$$\ell(P) = \sum_{i=1}^{m} w_i \log \sum_{j=1}^{k} p_j f(x_i, \lambda_j) = \sum_{i=1}^{m} w_i \log f(x_i, P). \qquad (4.22)$$

As a result, the log likelihood problem depends on P only through the possible values taken by the m-dimensional vector

$$\ell(P) = [\ell_1(P), \ell_2(P), \ldots, \ell_m(P)]^{\mathrm{T}}.$$

Now we change our perspective from maximizing the likelihood over all latent distributions P to the question of which of the eligible classes of mixture likelihood vectors $\ell(P)$ gives the largest value for the log likelihood. In other words we cast our problem into an optimization problem. In the first step the feasible region is constructed. Here the feasible region is given by the set $\Omega = \{\ell(P)|P$ is a distribution with finite support$\}$. In the next step the objective function is defined. The problem of maximizing $\ell(P)$ over all distributions P can be written as the problem of maximizing the objective function

$$\ell(p) := \sum_{i=1}^{m} w_i \log p_i$$

over the elements $p = (p_1, p_2, \ldots, p_m)^{\mathrm{T}}$ in the set Ω. Now the set Ω is convex and the objective function is concave; thus, convex optimization theory can be applied to find the maximum likelihood solution. First the set Ω is described. Consider the m-dimensional set Γ of all possible likelihood kernels that could arise from a degenerate one-component mixing distribution

$$\Gamma = \{f(x_1, \lambda), f(x_2, \lambda), \ldots, f(x_m, \lambda) | \lambda \in \Lambda\}.$$

The convex hull of Γ, i.e., the set of all convex combinations of Γ is $\mathrm{co}[\Gamma]$, is denoted as

$$\mathrm{co}[\Gamma] = \left\{ \sum_i p_i f_i(x_i, \lambda) | f_i \in \Gamma, p_i \geq 0, \sum p_i = 1 \right\}.$$

If the unicomponent likelihood curve is defined as $\Gamma = \{L(\lambda) | \lambda \in \Lambda\}$, then it follows that $\mathrm{co}[\Gamma]$ is also the set Ω. Thus, the elements of Γ can be thought of as a basis such as that all eligible mixture vectors are convex combinations from this basic set.

Now if Γ is closed and bounded, then $\mathrm{co}(\Gamma)$ is a compact subset of $\mathbb{R}^m$ and also closed and bounded. This guarantees that the continuous function $f(\phi) = \sum w_i \log f_i$ obtains its maximum on $\mathrm{co}(\Gamma)$. Following from Theorem 4.2, it is unique. According to the theorem of Carathéodory (Therorem 4.1) the solution has no more than m points of support, since the solution is on the boundary of the convex hull. This is summarized in Theorem 18 of Lindsay (1995).

Theorem 4.5.

1. *Suppose that* $\mathrm{co}(\Gamma)$ *is closed and bounded and that* Ω *contains at least one point with positive likelihood. Then there exists a unique* $\hat{P} \in \partial \Omega$ *the boundary of* Ω, *such that* $\hat{P}$ *maximizes* $\ell(p)$ *over* Ω.
2. *The associated* $\hat{P}$ *has at most m points of support.*

Example 4.3. Consider a random sample of size two from a mixture of normal component densities with unknown means λ_j and variances equal to 1 and $x_1 = 1.5$ and $x_2 = 2.5$. Then the curve Γ has the form

$$\Gamma = \left\{ \frac{1}{\sqrt{2\pi}} \exp\left[-\frac{(1.5 - \lambda)^2}{2} \right], \frac{1}{\sqrt{2\pi}} \exp\left[-\frac{(2.5 - \lambda)^2}{2} \right] | \lambda \in \Lambda \right\}.$$

Figure 4.12 shows the set Γ as a solid line and $\mathrm{co}[\Gamma]$ is the convex region inside the boundary of $\mathrm{co}[\Gamma]$. The dashed lines are contours of the objective function $\ell(p)$. The point marked with an asterisk on the boundary of $\mathrm{co}[\Gamma]$ is the point that maximizes the log likelihood.

This geometric characterization has moved us closer to a solution. One strategy to find a solution would be to maximize the likelihood over k components each k less or equal to m and then to choose the number of components with the largest

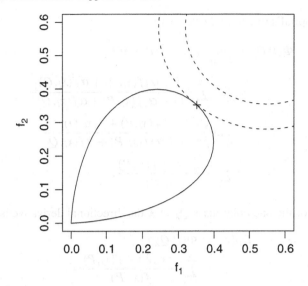

Fig. 4.12 The *solid line* is the curve Γ for two observations ($x_1 = 1.5$; $x_2 = 2.5$) from normal component densities with variances equal to one. The *region within the solid curve* is co$[\Gamma]$. The *dotted lines* show the contours of the log likelihood. The point marked with a *plus* is the point p_1, p_2 at which the likelihood is maximized, subject to the constraint that $p_1, p_2 \in$ co$[\Gamma]$

likelihood. Of course, this is still computationally expensive and it would be difficult to decide whether the global maximum has been attained.

The Directional Derivative

Fortunately the optimal solution $\hat{P}$ can be characterized in terms of directional derivatives. They are the major tool for obtaining characterizations and algorithms for the flexible support size case, where P and Q are probability measures with finite support. For $\alpha \in [0, 1]$ we define

$$\ell^*(\alpha) := \ell((1-\alpha)P + \alpha Q) = \sum_{i=1}^{n} \log f(x_i, (1-\alpha)P + \alpha Q)$$

$$= \sum_{i=1}^{n} \log\big((1-\alpha)f(x_i, P) + \alpha f(x_i, Q)\big).$$

(4.23)

Taking the derivative of $\ell^*(\alpha)$ at $\alpha = 0$ gives

$$\Phi(P, Q) = \lim_{\alpha \to 0} \frac{\ell((1-\alpha)P + \alpha Q) - \ell(P)}{\alpha}.$$

(4.24)

Applying l'Hôpital's rule to (4.24) leads to

$$
\begin{aligned}
\Phi(P,Q) &= \lim_{\alpha \to 0} [\ell((1-\alpha)P + \alpha Q)]' \\
&= \lim_{\alpha \to 0} \sum_{i=1}^{n} \frac{[(1-\alpha)f(x_i,P) + \alpha f(x_i,Q)]'}{(1-\alpha)f(x_i,P) + \alpha f(x_i,Q)} \\
&= \lim_{\alpha \to 0} \sum_{i=1}^{n} \frac{-f(x_i,P) + f(x_i,Q)}{(1-\alpha)f(x_i,P) + \alpha f(x_i,Q)} \\
&= \sum_{i=1}^{n} \frac{f(x_i,Q) - f(x_i,P)}{f(x_i,P)}.
\end{aligned}
\tag{4.25}
$$

In particular, for the one point mass Q_λ at λ the directional derivative is given by

$$
\begin{aligned}
D_P(\lambda) &= \Phi(P,Q_\lambda) \\
&= \sum_{i=1}^{n} \frac{f(x_i,\lambda) - f(x_i,P)}{f(x_i,P)} \\
&= \sum_{i=1}^{n} \frac{f(x_i,\lambda)}{f(x_i,P)} - n \\
&= \sum_{i=1}^{n} \frac{f(x_i,\lambda)}{\sum_{l=1}^{k} p_l f(x_i,\lambda_l)} - n.
\end{aligned}
\tag{4.26}
$$

The determining part in this directional derivative, namely, $\frac{1}{n}\sum_{i=1}^{n} \frac{f(x_i,\lambda)}{f(x_i,P)}$, is called the gradient function and is denoted by $d(\lambda,P)$.

Example 4.4. For the Poisson distribution the gradient function is given by

$$
d(\lambda,P) = \frac{1}{n} \sum_{i=1}^{n} \frac{e^{-\lambda}\lambda^{x_i}}{\sum_j p_j e^{-\lambda_j} \lambda_j^{x_i}}.
$$

Now, the general mixture maximum likelihood theorem states

Theorem 4.6.

1. *$\hat{P}$ is discrete and has at most n support points λ.*
2. *$\hat{P}$ is the NPMLE if and only if $D_P(\lambda) \leq 0 \; \forall \lambda$ or*
   $\frac{1}{n}\sum_{i=1}^{n} \frac{f(x_i,\lambda)}{f(x_i,P)} \leq 1 \; \forall \lambda$, respectively.
3. *$D_P(\lambda) = 0$ for all support points of $\hat{P}$.*
4. *The final part is that the fitted values of the likelihood, namely,*

$$
L(\hat{Q}) = (L_1(\hat{Q}), \ldots, L_n(\hat{Q})),
$$

are uniquely determined. That is, even if there were two distributions maximizing the likelihood, they would generate the same likelihood.

Details and proofs may be found in the monographs of Lindsay (1995) and Böhning (1999b) .

4.3.2 Algorithms for Flexible Support Size

The concept of directional derivatives is important in developing reliable converging algorithms; see Böhning (1995) and Lindsay and Lesperance (1995) for a review. Here we present only the basic ideas of two algorithms for the flexible support size case. The first one is the *vertex direction method* (VDM). This method is based on the following property of the directional derivative $D_P(\lambda)$: If $D_P(\lambda^+) > 0$ for some λ^+, then the likelihood can be increased over $\ell(P)$ by using a distribution with additional mass at λ^+. Formally there exists an α such that

$$\ell((1 - \alpha)P + \alpha Q_\lambda^+) > \ell(P), \qquad (4.27)$$

where Q_λ^+ is a distribution with mass 1 at λ. Hence, the VDM first chooses λ^+ to maximize $D_P(\lambda)$ and then maximizes over α in the one-parameter family $(1 - \alpha)P + \alpha Q_\lambda^+$. The maximization over α has no explicit solution and requires a secondary univariate algorithm. The parameter α may be seen as a step-length parameter. This leads to the following algorithm: The VDM is a natural algorithm to

---

Let P_0 be any initial value
Step 1: Find $\lambda_{\max}$ such that $D_P(\lambda_{\max}) = \sup_\lambda D_P(\lambda)$
Step 2: Find $\alpha_{\max}$ such that
$\ell((1 - \alpha_{\max})P^{(l)} + \alpha_{\max} Q_{\lambda^{\max}}) = \sup_\alpha \ell((1 - \alpha_{\max})P^{(l)} + \alpha_{\max} Q_{\lambda^{\max}})$
Step 3: Set $P^{(l+1)} = (1 - \alpha_{\max})P^{(l)} + \alpha_{\max} Q_{\lambda^{\max}}$, l=l+1 and go to step 1

Algorithm 4.3.1: Vertex direction method

---

compute the NPMLE. However, it may be painfully slow and thus a faster algorithm is desirable. One faster algorithm available is the vertex exchange method. The basic idea is as follows. If λ^+ maximizes $D_P(\lambda)$ and λ^- minimizes $D_P(\lambda)$, it is possible to increase the likelihood by adding more mass to λ^+ and subtracting mass from λ^-. Thus, the algorithm first chooses λ^+ and λ^-. Then we maximize the likelihood (or at least ensure monotonic increase) by incorporating a step α in a one-parameter family that exchanges the mass between λ^+ and λ^-: $P + \alpha P(\lambda^-)(Q_{\lambda+} - Q_{\lambda-})$, where Q_λ is again a distribution with mass 1 at λ. Clearly, if $\alpha = 1$ the "bad" support point λ^- is exchanged with the "good" support point λ^+. Thus, we have the following algorithm:

Let P_0 be any initial value
Step 1: Find $\lambda_{\max}$ such that $D_P(\lambda_{\max}) = \sup_\lambda D_P(\lambda)$ and find $\lambda_{\min}$ such that $D_P(\lambda_{\min}) = \min(D_P(\lambda)|\lambda \in$ support of $P^{(l)})$
Step 2: Find $\alpha_{\max}$ such that
$\ell(P^{(l)} + \alpha P^{(l)}(\lambda^-)(Q_{\lambda+} - Q_{\lambda-})) = \sup_\alpha \ell(P^{(l)} + \alpha P^{(l)}(\lambda^-)(Q_{\lambda+} - Q_{\lambda-}))$
Step 3: Set $P^{(l+1)} = P^{(l)} + \alpha_{\max} P^{(l)}(\lambda^-)(Q_{\lambda+} - Q_{\lambda-})$, $l = l+1$ and go to step 1

Algorithm 4.3.2: Vertex exchange method (VEM) algorithm

4.3.3 VEM Algorithm: Computation

Example: Vitamin A Supplementation and Childhood Mortality

Supplementation of vitamins is not only supposed to be beneficial for the prevention of cancer as discussed in Sect. 2.1. Fawzi et al. (1993) study the effect of vitamin A supplementation and childhood mortality in preschool children. They concluded that vitamin A supplements are associated with a significant reduction in mortality when given periodically to children at the community level.

These data were also used by Böhning (2003) and we will reproduce this author's calculations in this example. The data are listed in Table 4.1. All studies were community randomized trials from South Asia or Southeast Asia, except the second study, which was from northern Sudan. The incidence density was estimated according to $ID = E/T$, where E is the number of child deaths and T denotes the person time. The latter is calculated as the product of the number of children at risk and the number of years of observation. Hence, the rate ratio (RR) was estimated as $RR = \frac{ID_A}{ID_C}$. The index refers to intervention with vitamin A supplementation (A) or to the control group (C). The variance of $\log(RR)$ is estimated as $\text{var}(\log(RR)) = 1/E_A + 1/E_C$, with the indices as previously defined. The question is whether vitamin A supplementation is beneficial and whether the effect is more beneficial in some studies than in others. Apparently, there is heterogeneity of treatment effects $x_i = \log(RR)$, which can be modeled using a finite mixture model $f(x_i) = p_1 f(x_i, \theta_1) + \cdots + f(x_i, \theta_k)$, where $f(x_i, \theta) = N(x_i, \theta, \sigma_i)$ is the normal density with mean θ and variance σ_i^2. This is the variance as provided in the last column of Table 4.1. Thus, we are dealing with a meta-analysis, as described in detail in Chap. 7. As outlined there, a key point of any meta-analysis is the analysis of heterogeneity. A natural tool to do this is the application of finite mixture models as described in Sect. 7.3.

Table 4.1 Meta-analysis of mortality in community-based trials of vitamin A supplementation in children aged 6–72 months (cases; population)

Location	Observation time	Vitamin A	Control	log (RR)	Variance
Sarlahi (Nepal)	12	152; 14,487	210; 14,143	−0.34726	0.011341
Northern Sudan	18	123; 14,446	117; 14,294	0.03943	0.016677
Tamil Nadu (India)	12	37; 7,764	80; 7,655	−0.78525	0.039527
Aceh (Indonesia)	12	101; 12,991	130; 12,209	−0.31450	0.017593
Hyderabad (India)	12	39; 7,691	41; 8,084	−0.00017	0.050031
Jumla (Nepal)	5	138; 3,786	167; 3,411	−0.29504	0.013234
Java (Indonesia)	12	186; 5,775	250; 5,445	−0.35455	0.009376
Mumbai (India)	42	7; 1,784	32; 1,644	−1.60155	0.174107

RR rate ratio

VEM Algorithm

We begin our analysis with the application of the VEM algorithm. First, we need to load the library CAMAN and the data set *vitA*. This is done by typing

```
> library(CAMAN)
> data(vitA)
```

The first choice in using the VEM algorithm for the flexible support size involves the selection of a grid of parameter values $\theta_1, \ldots, \theta_m$ over which we wish to find the corresponding population proportions that maximize the likelihood function. The default in *mixalg.VEM* calculates the minimum and the maximum of the data and constructs a grid with $k = 25$ equidistant grid points. Here we use a grid of 20 points. Now, the VEM algorithm is used as follows:

```
> m0<-mixalg.VEM(obs="logrr",var.lnOR="var",
  family="gaussian",data=vitA,startk=20)
```

The algorithm identified four grid points with positive weight. These are shown by typing

```
> m0

Computer Assisted Mixture Analysis (VEM):

Data consist of 8 observations (rows)

4 grid points with positive support

p    parameter
.0994      -1.600000
.1175      -.823158
.6189      -.305263
.1643       .040000

Log-Likelihood:-1.27124
```

A plot of the grid point θ versus the gradient function $d(\theta, P)$ is obtained as follows:

```
> plot(m0@totalgrid[,2],m0@totalgrid[,3],
type="l",xlab="parameter",ylab="gradient")
```

This plot is shown in Fig. 4.13. Note that in this plot the gradient function takes the value unity if there is a positive weight.

We proceed with a discussion of the expectation maximization (EM) algorithm, which assumes the number of components k to be known, i.e., the fixed support size case.

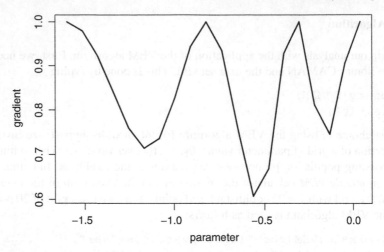

Fig. 4.13 Parameter θ versus gradient function $d(\theta, P)$

4.4 The Fixed Support Size Case

4.4.1 Fixed Support Size: The Newton–Raphson Algorithm

Also in the fixed support size case maximum likelihood estimation of P is by no means trivial, since again there are mostly no closed-form solutions available. One of the frequently used iterative methods in maximum likelihood estimation is the Newton–Raphson (NR) method.

This algorithm maximizes the log likelihood:

$$\ell(P) = \log L(P) = \sum_{i=1}^{n} \log \sum_{j=1}^{k} f(x_i, \lambda_j) p_j. \tag{4.28}$$

The NR method solves the likelihood equation for a fixed number of components k

$$S(x, P) = 0 \tag{4.29}$$

by approximating the gradient vector $S(x, P)$ of the log likelihood function $\ell(P)$ by a linear Taylor series expansion about the current fit $P^{(l)}$ for P. This approach gives

$$S(x, P) \approx S(x, P^{(l)}) - I(x, P^{(l)})(P - P^{(l)}), \tag{4.30}$$

where $I(x, P)$ is the information matrix. A new fit $P^{(l+1)}$ is obtained by equating $S(x, P)$ of the right-hand side to zero and solving for $P^{(l+1)}$:

$$P^{(l+1)} = P^{(l)} - I^{-1}(x, P^{(l)}) S(x, P^{(l)}). \tag{4.31}$$

The NR algorithm converges quadratically, which is very fast and is regarded as a major strength of the algorithm. Everitt (1984) compared several algorithms for the estimation of the parameters of a mixture of two normals and found the NR algorithm to be the fastest. But there can be potentially severe problems in applications. First the algorithm requires at each iteration the computation of the inverse of the $d \times d$ information matrix $I(x, P^{(l)})$ and the solution of a system of d linear equations. Thus, the computation required for an iteration is likely to become expensive when d is large. Also one must allow for the storage of the Hessian or some set of factors of it. Second, for some applications the algorithm also requires an impractically accurate guess of P for the sequence of iterates $P^{(l)}$ to converge to the global maximum. For the mixture problem at hand there is no guarantee that the algorithm will converge from any arbitrary starting value. Titterington et al. (1985) demonstrated for mixtures of normals divergence of the algorithm depending on the starting values. Another difficulty lies in the fact that besides initial values for the parameters also the number of components k needs to be fixed in advance.

4.4.2 A General Description of the EM Algorithm

For the fixed support size case the maximum likelihood procedures for the estimation of the parameters rely on the use of the EM algorithm (Dempster et al. 1977; Aitkin and Wilson 1980; Redner and Walker 1984; Aitkin and Rubin 1985). A detailed overview of the theory and applications of the EM algorithm may be found in the monographs of McLachlan and Krishnan (1997) and Watanabe and Yamaguchi (2004). The application and modification of the EM algorithm for finite mixtures is still an active area of research. Recent developments and modifications of the EM algorithm in the mixture framework are given, for example, in the articles by Pilla and Lindsay (2001), Vlassis and Likas (2002), Arcidiacono and Jones (2003), and Verbeek et al. (2006). The EM algorithm, in general, requires a particular model structure. The key idea of the EM algorithm is data augmentation. Suppose that we have in our model with parameters Ψ both observed data X and missing data Z. We need to maximize the likelihood of the observed data X, labeled $L_X(\Psi)$, this likelihood is difficult to maximize, as for example in the mixture setting. If we assume that we know the unobserved data Z, then the maximization of the *complete* data likelihood $L_c(\Psi) = L_{X,Z}(\Psi)$ of the pair (X, Z) would be easy. In the ideal case it would have explicit solutions. For the application of the algorithm the "missing data" may be completely imaginary. The important idea is that the distribution of the variable X is the same as the marginal distribution of X in some hypothetical pair X, Z which has an easier to deal with likelihood.

The E-step in the EM algorithm involves taking a current value $\Psi^{(0)}$ and finding $Q(\Psi; \Psi^{(0)})$, which is the conditional expectation of the full data log likelihood $\log L_c(\Psi)$ given the observed data

$$Q(\Psi; \Psi^{(0)}) = E_{\Psi^{(0)}} \left[\log L_c(\Psi \mid x) \right]. \tag{4.32}$$

The M-step then requires the maximization of $Q(\Psi; \Psi^{(0)})$ with respect to Ψ over the parameter space Ω. This implies choosing $\Psi^{(1)}$ such that

$$Q(\Psi^{(1)}; \Psi^{(0)}) \geq Q(\Psi; \Psi^{(0)}), \quad \forall \Psi \in \Omega. \tag{4.33}$$

The E-step and the M-step are then carried out again with $\Psi^{(0)}$ replaced by the current fit $\Psi^{(1)}$. On the $(l+1)$th iteration the E-step and the M-step are defined as follows:

E-step: Calculate $Q(\Psi; \Psi^{(l)})$ with

$$Q(\Psi; \Psi^{(l)}) = E_{\Psi^{(l)}} [\log L_c(\Psi \mid x)]. \tag{4.34}$$

M-step: Choose $\Psi^{(l+1)}$ to be any value of $\Psi \in \Omega$ that maximizes $\Psi^{(l)}$:

$$Q(\Psi^{(l+1)}; \Psi^{(l)}) \geq Q(\Psi; \Psi^{(l)}). \tag{4.35}$$

Detailed investigations of the convergence properties of the EM algorithm may be found in Dempster et al. (1977), Wu (1983), and McLachlan and Krishnan (1997).

4.4.3 The EM Algorithm for Finite Mixture Models

In the mixture model setting we treat the component membership as the missing data. Thus, we have the observed data X and the unknown indicator variable Z which indicates the membership of the ith observation in the jth component. Let $z_{ij} \in \{0, 1\}$ denote the value of Z_j for observation x_i. The likelihood for the pair $(x_i, z_{i1}, \dots, z_{ik})^T$ is

$$\Pr(X_i = x_i, Z_{i1} = z_{i1}, \dots, Z_{ik} = z_{ik})$$
$$= \Pr(X_i = x_i \mid Z_{i1} = z_{i1}, \dots, Z_{ik} = z_{ik})\Pr(Z_{i1} = z_{i1}, \dots, Z_{ik} = z_{ik})$$
$$= \prod_{j=1}^{k} p_i^{z_{ij}} f(x_i, \lambda_j)^{z_{ij}}.$$

Hence, the likelihood is as follows

$$L_c(P) = \prod_{i=1}^{n} \prod_{j=1}^{k} p_i^{z_{ij}} f(x_i, \lambda_j)^{z_{ij}}. \tag{4.36}$$

The complete data log likelihood is given by

$$\log L_c(P) = \sum_{i=1}^{n} \sum_{j=1}^{k} z_{ij} \log p_i + \sum_{i=1}^{n} \sum_{j=1}^{k} z_{ij} \log f(x_i, \lambda_j). \tag{4.37}$$

To perform the E-step of the EM algorithm we replace the z_{ij} with their expected values given the data $x_1, \ldots, x_n$. Applying Bayes's theorem, we obtain

$$\Pr(Z_{ij} = 1 \mid X_i = x_i) = \frac{\Pr(X_i = x_i \mid Z_{ij} = 1)\Pr(Z_{ij} = 1)}{\sum_l \Pr(X_i = x_i \mid Z_{il} = 1)\Pr(Z_{il} = 1)}$$

$$= \frac{p_j f(x_i, \lambda_j)}{\sum_l p_l f(x_i, \lambda_l)} := e_{ij}. \qquad (4.38)$$

Hence, replacing z_{ij} with e_{ij} in (4.37) leads to

$$Q(P, P^{(l)}) = E_{P^{(l)}}(\log L_c(P))$$

$$= \sum_{i=1}^{n} \sum_{j=1}^{k} e_{ij} \log p_j + \sum_{i=1}^{n} \sum_{j=1}^{k} e_{ij} \log f(x_i, \lambda_j). \qquad (4.39)$$

This is the E-step in a mixture model. The M-step involves maximization of the current expected complete data likelihood. Since p_j appears only in the left term, and λ_j only in the right term, we can maximize the two terms separately. For the mixing weights this simply involves

$$p_j^{(l+1)} = \frac{\sum_i e_{ij}}{n} = \sum_i \frac{p_j f(x_i, \lambda_j)}{\sum_l p_l f(x_i, \lambda_l)} / n. \qquad (4.40)$$

If the component parameters are unknown, they are estimated by finding the maximum likelihood estimator for the second sum of the expected complete data likelihood. In the Poisson case this gives

$$\lambda_j^{(l+1)} = \frac{\sum_i e_{ij} x_i}{\sum_i e_{ij}}. \qquad (4.41)$$

Now, let us consider the normal density

$$f(x, \lambda_j) = \frac{1}{\sqrt{2\pi\sigma^2}} e^{-\frac{(x-\lambda_j)^2}{2\sigma^2}}. \qquad (4.42)$$

Again, $\lambda_j^{(l+1)}$ is given by (4.41). Taking the derivative of (4.37) with respect to σ^2 leads to the likelihood equation

$$\sum_{i=1}^{n} \sum_{j=1}^{k} e_{ij}(x_i - \lambda_j)^2 / \sigma^4 + \sum_{i=1}^{n} \sum_{j=1}^{k} e_{ij} / \sigma^2.$$

This likelihood equation has the solution

$$\sigma_{l+1}^2 = \frac{1}{n} \sum_{i=1}^{n} \sum_{j=1}^{k} e_{ij}(x_i - \lambda_j)^2. \qquad (4.43)$$

Note that we assume a common variance for all components. The reason for this is the well-known degeneracy of the likelihood function for component-specific variances σ_j^2. Nityasuddhi and Böhning (2003) investigated the EM algorithm to find estimators of the normal mixture distribution with unknown component specific variances and identify situations in which the EM algorithm works in that case. Ridolfi and Idier (1999) proposed applying penalized maximum likelihood to circumvent the problem. In summary, the EM algorithm for the fixed support size case is given as

---

Step 0: Let P be any vector of starting values
Step 1: Compute the E-step according to (4.38)
Step 2: Compute the M-step according to (4.40) and (4.41), leading to $P^{(l)}$ and $\lambda^{(l)}$
Step 3: Let $P=P^{(l)}$ and go to step 1

Algorithm 4.4.1: Expectation maximization (EM) algorithm

One major advantage of the EM algorithm is given by the fact that it always converges, but with the disadvantage that it converges to a local maximum. Another disadvantage of the EM algorithm is its sometimes very slow convergence. Thus, there have been many attempts to accelerate the speed of convergence. The most commonly used method is the multivariate Aitken acceleration (Louis 1982). Other attempts to accelerate the EM algorithm are based on quasi-Newton methods (Meilijson 1989; Jamshidian and Jennrich 1993, 1997; Lange 1995). These methods require some convergence diagnostics and do not keep the simplicity of the EM algorithm. Another line of research tries to conserve the simplicity of the EM algorithm by using different methods of data augmentation. These ideas are presented in the articles by Meng and Rubin (1993) and Liu and Rubin (1994). An overview of these methods may be found in the paper by Meng and van Dyk (1997). More recently Ng and McLachlan (2004) showed how a modified EM algorithm can be sped up by adopting a multiresolution kd-tree structure in performing the E-step. Several authors have published program code for the estimation of the parameters of a mixture model using the EM algorithm; see, for example, Agha and Ibrahim (1984), Agha and Branker (1997), and DerSimonian (1986). Jones and McLachlan (1990) provided Fortran code for mixtures of grouped and truncated mixtures of normals. The EM algorithm is implemented in the programs C.A.MAN (Böhning et al. 1992, 1998) and DismapWin (Schlattmann et al. 1996) as well. Schlattmann et al. (2003) developed the program META, which provides mixture model estimation in the context of meta-analysis. See also Chap. 7 for an application of mixture models in this field. Recently Biernacki et al. (2006) introduced the MIXMOD program for model-based discrimination and clustering. Proust and Jacqmin-Gadda (2005) applied the EM algorithm in their program HETMIXLIN which extends the method to linear mixed models for longitudinal data. Finite mixture models for longitudinal data are also discussed in Sect. 4.7, where this type of model is fit to pharmacokinetic data. The choice of starting values is crucial when applying the EM algorithm (Karlis and Xekalaki 2003). Depending on the starting values, the algorithm may converge to a local rather than to a global maximum. Laird (1978) suggested a grid search, which leads to a large number of parameters. McLachlan and Basford (1988, Sect. 1.7) suggested first applying a clustering algorithm and using this result as starting values for the EM algorithm. More recently Biernacki et al. (2003) and Biernacki (2004) proposed the use of the stochastic EM algorithm (Celeux et al. 1996), which at each EM iteration selects new random weights p_j. Dias and Wedel (2004) found in a simulation study that this algorithm is superior to the EM algorithm. A disadvantage of this procedure lies in the fact it does not converge pointwise. Berchtold (2004) found by simulation that two-stage procedures combining both an exploration phase and an optimization phase provide the best results, especially when these methods are applied on several sets of initial conditions rather than on one single starting point. One such hybrid procedure is the following algorithm proposed and developed by the author of this monograph. Before we introduce this algorithm, we present in the next section the use of the R package CAMAN with regard to the EM algorithm.

4.4.4 EM Algorithm: Computation

Coming back to our example on vitamin A supplementation and childhood mortality on page 70, we now fit various models using the EM algorithm. The simplest one is the homogenous model, which states that all studies find the same effect. This model is fit using the following code:

```
> m1<-mixalg.EM(obs="logrr",var.lnOR="var",
family="gaussian",p=c(1),t=c(0),data=vitA)
```

Here, the function *mixalg.EM* is called with starting values for a single component. This implicitly indicates that k is set equal to unity.

Typing *m1* shows the shortened results of this model:

```
> m1


   p       mean
1  1  -0.3087638


Log-Likelihood: -5.003965      BIC: 12.08737
```

Obviously, the log likelihood is worse than that obtained with the VEM algorithm, which was -1.271. Thus, next a model with two components is fit to the data. Here we give equal weight to -1.6 and -0.5 as starting values. This is done using the following code:

```
> m2<-mixalg.EM(obs="logrr",var.lnOR="var",
family="gaussian",p=c(0.5,0.5),t=c(-1.6,-0.5),
data=vitA)
```

The result is obtained as

```
> m2
```

```
           p         mean
1  0.1186638  -1.5990254
2  0.8813362  -0.2924686
```

```
Log-Likelihood: -3.103066      BIC: 12.44446
```

In terms of the Bayesian information criterion (BIC) defined as $\text{BIC} = -2\ell(P) + (2k-1) + \log(n)$ this model is only slightly better than a homogenous model. But, as mentioned before, the EM algorithm may converge to a local maximum and it is thus recommended to use several different starting values. The next model gives equal weight to -0.5 and 0 as starting values. The call to the function is then

```
> m3<-mixalg.EM(obs="logrr",var.lnOR="var",
family="gaussian",p=c(0.5,0.5),t=c(-0.5,0),data=vitA)
```

This gives the result

```
> m3
```

```
DETAILS:
           p         mean
1  0.8170025  -0.37132965
2  0.1829975   0.02792931
```

```
Log-Likelihood: -3.237008      BIC: 12.71234
```

This model is even worse. The next set of starting values is given by equal weights to -1.6 and 0.

```
> m4<-mixalg.EM(obs="logrr",var.lnOR="var",
family="gaussian",p=c(0.5,0.5),t=c(-1.6,0),data=vitA)
```

This leads to the result

```
> m4
           p         mean
1  0.2245207  -0.9462519
2  0.7754793  -0.2666073
```

```
Log-Likelihood: -2.730582      BIC: 11.69949
```

On the basis of this result, the model *m4* with $k = 2$ components would be chosen according to the BIC. However, the likelihood of the flexible support size model was better, i.e., equal to 1.271.

In terms of interpretation, a beneficial effect of vitamin A supplementation is revealed, but this effect is certainly heterogeneous. It would be interesting to identify the determinants of this heterogeneity.

It seems natural to combine the EM and VEM algorithms to start the EM algorithm with starting values at the global maximum provided by the VEM algorithm.

4.4.5 A Hybrid Mixture Algorithm

This hybrid mixture algorithm (Algorithm 4.4.2) proposed by Schlattmann (2003) combines the VEM algorithm (Algorithm 4.3.2) for flexible support size and the EM algorithm (Algorithm 4.4.1). The solution of the VEM algorithm provides starting values for the EM algorithm. By the NPMLE theorem, the EM algorithm thus starts very close to the global maximum and proper convergence of the EM algorithm to a global maximum is ensured. This sequential algorithm leads to an initial estimate of the NPMLE and a proper solution for the subsequent EM algorithm. Crucial points are the definitions of δ and ε. Depending on these settings, different solutions could result from this algorithm.

Step 1: Define an approximating grid $\lambda_1, \ldots, \lambda_L$
Step 2: Use the VEM algorithm to maximize $L(P)$ in the simplex Ω_{grid} and identify grid points with positive support. Here positive support is defined as $p_j \geq \varepsilon$ (often $\varepsilon = 10^{-2}$), $j = 1, \ldots, L$.
This gives an initial estimate of $\hat{k}$
Step 3: Use these $\hat{k}$ points and corresponding mixing weights p_j as starting values for the EM algorithm
Step 4: Collapse identical components if $| \lambda_j - \lambda_i | < \delta$ (often $\delta = 0.05$) $\quad i \neq j$
Step 5: Obtain the final number of components $\hat{k}$

Algorithm 4.4.2: A mixture algorithm combining the VEM and EM algorithms

---

Computation

This hybrid algorithm is called as follows:

```
> m5<-mixalg(obs="logrr",var.lnOR="var",
family="gaussian",data=vitA,startk=20)
```

This gives the result

```
> m5
Computer Assisted Mixture Analysis:

Data consist of 8 observations (rows).
The Mixture Analysis identified 4 components
```

```
DETAILS:
                p            mean
1  0.1004267  -1.60088222
2  0.1066273  -0.82222330
3  0.6157952  -0.32872949
4  0.1771508   0.02822363


Log-Likelihood: -1.195960      BIC: 16.94801
```

This model has four components with a log likelihood of -1.19. In terms of the BIC this model is worse than the two-component model identified previously. This is due to the large number of parameters.

An alternative algorithm which applies the information given by the gradient within the framework of the EM algorithm is described in the next section.

4.4.6 The EM Algorithm with Gradient Update

Another algorithm to improve the behavior of the EM algorithm proposed by Böhning (2003) applies a combination of gradient function steps and EM steps to achieve global convergence. More specifically, the general mixture maximum likelihood theorem (Theorem 4.6) states that $\hat{P}$ is the NPMLE if and only if the directional derivative $\Phi(P,Q_\lambda) \leq 0$ for all λ or alternatively if the gradient function $\sum_{i=1}^{n} \frac{f(x_i,\lambda)}{\sum_{j=1}^{k} p_j f(x_i,\lambda_j)} - n$ is equal to unity.

Thus, a natural extension of the EM algorithm incorporates the information provided by the gradient as described in Algorithm 4.4.3. Coming back to our example

---

Step 0: Let P be any vector of starting values
Step 1: Use the EM algorithm to estimate $\hat{P}_{EM}$
Step 2: Determine λ_{max} to maximize $d(\lambda, \hat{P}_{EM})$
Step 3: Determine λ_{min} such that
$\ell(P_{EM} + P_{EM}(\lambda_j)[Q_{max} - Q_{min}] | j = 1,\ldots,k)$ is largest
Step 5: Exchange λ_{max} with λ_{min}. Go to step 2

Algorithm 4.4.3: EM algorithm with gradient update

dealing with vitamin A supplementation, we saw that different starting values for the EM algorithm led to different log likelihoods. Owing to different likelihoods, different values of the BIC were obtained. As a result, depending on the starting values, different conclusions with regard to the number components could be drawn.

The EM algorithm with gradient update circumvents these problems and gives the correct result. One of the key points in applying this algorithm is to find λ_{max} in step 2 of the algorithm. Figure 4.14 shows a plot of the parameter λ

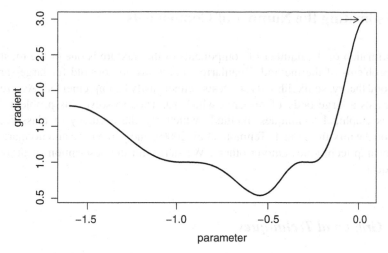

Fig. 4.14 Gradient function $d(\lambda, P)$ versus λ, with $\lambda \in [-1.6, 0.4]$

versus the gradient function after step 1 of Algorithm 4.4.3. The arrow indicates $\lambda_{max} = 0.0377$, which is exchanged with λ_{min} in step 5 of the algorithm.

Note that in Algorithm 4.4.3 the gradient is a scalar and the maximum of the gradient can easily be found on a grid or by a line search. If a vector of parameters is to be found as in regression models, finding λ_{max} may be more complicated. This problem is addressed in Sect. 4.6.4.

Computation

The EM algorithm with gradient update is used by setting the flag *gradup* = T in the call of the function *mixalg.EM*. In this case it is not necessary to define starting values; this is taken care of by the program.

```
> m6<-mixalg.EM(obs="logrr",var.lnOR="var",
family="gaussian",gradup=T,data=vitA)
```

This leads to the result

```
> m6
            p          mean
1 0.2245207 -0.9462519
2 0.7754793 -0.2666073

Log-Likelihood: -2.730582     BIC: 11.69949
```

Applying the EM algorithm with gradient update, one obtains the correct result.

4.5 Estimating the Number of Components

The estimation of the number of components of the mixture is one of the most difficult problems of the method. Regularity conditions do not hold for large-sample likelihood theory, so likelihood ratio tests cannot easily be implemented. As a result, there exists a large body of research which has tried to solve this problem. This includes graphical techniques, methods which use the accuracy of classification based on the mixture model (Tenmoto et al. 2000), and parametric and nonparametric bootstrap techniques among others. We start with the description of graphical techniques.

4.5.1 Graphical Techniques

The simplest way to estimate the number of components is to plot the empirical density of the data. If X is continuous, grouping the observations and counting the number of modes has to be considered. However, a mixture density is multimodal only under certain conditions and thus this approach may be quite insensitive. An overview of these techniques is given in the book by Everitt and Hand (1981); they also discuss conditions for mixtures of univariate normals to be multimodal. Inferential procedures for assessing the number of modes are given by Titterington et al. (1985, Sect. 5.6). Other approaches to assess the number of modes use kernel density estimates; see, for example, Silverman (1981). Efron and Tibshirani (1993, Sect. 16.5) considered bootstrap techniques to test the multimodality of a population. Roeder (1994) showed that a mixture of two normals divided by a normal density having the same mean and variance as the mixed density is always bimodal. A diagnostic technique which exploits the properties of the NPMLE was suggested by Lindsay and Roeder (1992). This approach focuses on the graphical analysis of the residuals

$$\frac{\text{Observed} - \text{expected}}{\text{expected}},$$

where "observed" is defined to be $w(y)$, the relative frequency of the sample elements equal to y. "Expected" is the expected frequency under the model considered; under the model $f(y, \lambda)$ we obtain the homogeneity residual $r_{\hat{\lambda}}(y) = \frac{w(y)}{f(y,\lambda)} - 1$, whereas $r_{\hat{P}}(y) = \frac{w(y)}{f(y,\hat{P})} - 1$ leads to the heterogeneity residuals. A certain pattern of homogeneity residuals plotted against the observations y can be indicative of a mixture model. This is very similar to regression diagnostics, where certain patterns are indicative of other models. Lindsay and Roeder (1992) have shown that a plot of $\log(r_{\hat{\lambda}}(y) + 1)$ should have a *convex* structure if a mixture model is present. See Fig. 3.2 on page 35 for an example.

4.5.2 Testing for the Number of Components

Frequently, it is necessary to test for the number of components of the mixture model. As before let $f(x, P_k) = f(x, \lambda_1)p_1 + \cdots + f(x, \lambda_k)p_k$ denote the mixture density. But now the number of components is explicitly indexed in $f(x, P_k)$. Thus, the log likelihood is given by $\ell(P) = \sum \log f(x_i, P_k)$.

We wish to test the following hypothesis

$$H_0 : \text{number of components} = k$$
$$\text{versus}$$
$$H_1 : \text{number of components} = k + 1$$

and make use of the LRS using the statistic (Cox and Hinkley 1974, p. 323)

$$\begin{aligned} \text{LRS} &= -2\log \xi_n \\ &= -2\left[\ell(\hat{P}_k) - \ell(\hat{P}_{k+1})\right]. \end{aligned} \tag{4.44}$$

An extensive discussion of the problem of likelihood ratio testing in mixture models may be found in the books by Titterington et al. (1985), McLachlan and Basford (1988), Lindsay (1995) , and Böhning (1999a). Aitkin and Rubin (1985) tried to overcome the problem of the irregular parameter space and to make the problem regular by using a prior distribution on the mixing weights p_j. However, Quinn et al. (1987) showed that even with this approach the regularity conditions are violated. Another way to establish regularity conditions was followed by Feng and McCulloch (1992). They showed that enlarging the parameter space leads to a classical asymptotic distribution. Chen (1998) obtained regularity by subtracting a penalty term from the log likelihood for a mixture of two binomials.

Goffinet et al. (1992) found the exact limiting distribution in several problems involving the normal distribution. Their results are based on the assumption that the mixing proportions are known a priori under the alternative, which in practice is hardly the case. Thus, in general, only little is known about the distribution of the LRS.

As a result, over the years many simulation studies have been performed to obtain the distribution of the LRS. Thode et al. (1988) performed a simulation study to test $k = 1$ compared with $k = 2$ for a mixture of two normals with an additional free and common variance parameter. They concluded that the distribution of the LRS is asymptotically χ^2 with two degrees of freedom, although convergence is slow. Mendell et al. (1991) considered the asymptotic distribution of $-2\log \xi_n$ under the *alternative hypothesis*. They conjectured that the asymptotic distribution could be noncentral χ^2 possibly with two degrees of freedom. Feng and McCulloch (1994) investigated the distribution for the LRS for mixtures of normals with unequal variance. Böhning et al. (1994) considered several densities from the one-parameter exponential family and found that the limiting distribution might be described by mixtures of χ^2 distributions. Atwood et al. (1996) did extensive simulations for the mixtures of normals. They concluded that although the asymptotic distribution is not a χ^2 distribution with two degrees of freedom, it does appear to be a good approximation to the upper 15% of the distribution (Fu et al. 2006).

Another idea in this setting is to include a penalty term such as Akaike's information criterion (AIC) or the BIC. This implies the introduction of penalty terms for the number of parameters estimated for the model at hand. An overview of the use of these criteria for model selection may be found in Carlin and Louis (1996). Leroux and Puterman (1992) applied these criteria in a mixture model setting. However, these criteria are useful in a model selection process, but they suffer from the same difficulties as the likelihood ratio test, i.e., violation of the regularity conditions. Polymenis and Titterington (1998) used an information-based eigenvalue that in theory becomes zero as soon as too many mixture components are included in the model. In a simulation exercise, their method appears to be equivalent to the bootstrap likelihood ratio method for large sample sizes Chen et al. (2001) proposed a modified LRS for homogeneity in finite mixture models with a general parametric kernel distribution family. The modified LRS has a χ^2 type of null limiting distribution and is asymptotically most powerful under local alternatives. The same authors (Chen et al. 2004) extended this approach to the problem of testing the hypothesis $k = 2$ compared with $k \geq 3$. Chen and Kalbfleisch (2005) incorporated a penalty term to avoid boundary problems. They considered the use of likelihood ratio results when an unknown structural parameter is involved in the model. They studied an application of the modified likelihood approach to finite normal mixture models with a common and unknown variance in the mixing components and considered a test of the hypothesis of a homogeneous model compared with a mixture on two or more components. They showed that the χ^2 distribution with two degrees of freedom has a stochastic lower bound to the limiting distribution of the LRS. Fu et al. (2006) applied the modified likelihood ratio test to two binomial mixture models arising in genetic linkage analysis. The limiting distribution of the test statistic for both models wass shown to be a mixture of χ^2 distributions. An overview of more recent asymptotic results in the problem of testing homogeneity against a two-component mixture was provided by Garel (2007).

Lo (2005) provided a discussion of the dependence of the rate of convergence of the LRS to its limiting distribution on the choice of restrictions imposed on the component variances to deal with the problem of unboundedness of the likelihood using simulation techniques. Susko (2003) introduced weighted versions of homogeneity tests that can be used to test for the presence of additional components in a mixture. Simulation studies performed suggest that the tests have power comparable to that of the bootstrap likelihood ratio test presented in the next section.

4.5.3 The Bootstrap Approach

All the results of the simulation studies mentioned before are more often than not difficult to apply to an individual data set. Aitkin et al. (1981) had reservations about the adequacy of χ^2 approximations for the null distribution of the LRS.

In the context of latent class analysis they approached the problem essentially using a bootstrap approach. The bootstrap was introduced by Efron (1979) and was investigated further in a series of articles. An overview is given in the book by Efron and Tibshirani (1993). A detailed overview of the theoretical properties of the bootstrap may be found in the book by Shao and Tu (1995). The bootstrap is a powerful technique that allows one to assess the variability in a random quantity using just the data at hand. An estimate $\hat{F}$ of the underlying distribution is obtained from the observed sample. Conditional on the latter, the sampling distribution of the quantity of interest with F replaced by $\hat{F}$ defines the bootstrap distribution. This bootstrap distribution is an approximation to the true distribution. An important feature is given by the fact that $\hat{F}$ is assumed to preserve the stochastic structure of the model. Usually there are no closed-form expressions available for the bootstrap distribution and they have to be approximated by Monte Carlo methods where (pseudo) random samples are drawn from $\hat{F}$. If the bootstrap is implemented *nonparametrically*, then it is based on the empirical distribution function of the data.

The Parametric Bootstrap To Estimate the Distribution of the LRS

To obtain the distribution of the LRS for the test of the null hypothesis $H_0 : k = k_1$ groups compared with $H_1 : k = k_2$ groups a *parametric* bootstrap can be applied as follows. Proceeding under H_0, one generates a bootstrap sample from a mixture of k_1 groups where unknown parameters are replaced by their likelihood estimates formed under H_0 from the original sample. The value of $2\log \xi_n$ defined in (4.44) is computed for the bootstrap sample after fitting mixture models with $k = k_1$ and $k = k_2$ components in turn. This process is repeated independently B times and the replicated values of $-2\log \xi_n$ formed by the successive bootstrap samples provide an assessment of the bootstrap and hence of the true null distribution of $2\log \xi_n$. Thus, it allows one to obtain an approximation to the achieved level of significance corresponding to the value of $-2\log \xi$ obtained from the original sample. The test which rejects H_0 if $-2\log \xi$ for the original data is larger than the jth smallest of its B bootstrap replications has size (Aitkin et al. 1981)

$$\alpha = 1 - \frac{j}{B+1}. \tag{4.45}$$

This approach is widely used to obtain the distribution of the LRS. See, for example, McLachlan et al. (1995), Karlis and Xekalaki (1999), and McLachlan and Khan (2004). A crucial point here is the number of bootstrap replications performed. An accurate result will require a large number of replications B. Efron and Tibshirani (1986) have shown that whereas for the estimation of a standard error 50–100 replications are sufficient, a larger number, say, 350, are necessary to obtain a useful estimate of a percentile or a p value.

The bootstrap simulation of the LRS is usually based on the EM algorithm. Seidel et al. (2000a) showed that different starting strategies and stopping rules yield completely different estimators of the model parameters. They demonstrated for the likelihood ratio test of homogeneity against two-component exponential mixtures that when the test statistic is calculated by the EM algorithm different critical values for the LRS may occur. As a result, statistical inference may be incorrect. Thus, alternatively nonparametric bootstrap methods were suggested and evaluated by Schlattmann (2003, 2005).

The Nonparametric Bootstrap Approach To Estimate the Number of Components k

Recently there has been growing interest in Bayesian methods for estimating the parameters of the mixture model. An overview may be found in Titterington et al. (1985) or Robert (1996). More recently the book by Frühwirth-Schnatter (2006)

Step 1: Sample B bootstrap samples and calculate $\hat{k}^{*^b}$, $b = 1, \ldots, B$ for each sample
Step 2: Estimate the number of components $\hat{k}_B$ using the mode of the B replications: $\hat{k}_B = $ argmax$f_B(\hat{k})$, where $f_B(\hat{k})$ is the frequency of the value $\hat{k}$ based on the B bootstrap replications

Algorithm 4.5.1: Nonparametric bootstrap algorithm to estimate k

---

covers Bayesian estimation of finite mixture models. These algorithms keep the number of components fixed. A Bayesian approach which does not need to keep the number of components fixed has been provided by Richardson and Green (1997). It makes use of reversible jump Markov chain Monte Carlo methods that are capable of jumping between the parameter subspaces corresponding to different numbers of components in the mixture. A sample from the full joint distribution of all unknown variables is thereby generated and this is used to investigate the posterior distribution of the number of components k. This approach does not require an initial estimate of the number of components k, but there is a need to define many prior distributions for the hyperparameters for this Bayesian setting.

In the discussion of this paper the nonparametric bootstrap approach was suggested by Schlattmann and Böhning (1997). Here the hybrid mixture algorithm was applied to bootstrap samples of the original data and repeated B times and hence the distribution of the number of components k was obtained.

Using the hybrid mixture algorithm (Algorithm 4.4.2) as outlined on page 79, we obtain an initial guess of the number of components k. If one is interested in the variability of k on empirical grounds, the bootstrap is a natural choice. Bootstrap methods depend on the notion of a bootstrap sample. This sample x^* is obtained from the original sample x with replacement. Corresponding to the bootstrap data set x^*, we obtain $\hat{k}^*$ by applying the mixture algorithm to the bootstrap sample. The bootstrap algorithm involves drawing B independent bootstrap samples and estimating $\hat{k}$ using the mixture algorithm. The result is the bootstrap distribution of the number of components $\hat{k}$. The stopping rule for both the VEM algorithm and the EM algorithm is given by $D_{P(l)}(\lambda_{\max}) < \varepsilon$, where $\varepsilon = 10^{-7}$. The maximum number of iterations is 10,000. The use of the VEM algorithm, which according to Theorem 4.6 provides the global maximum of the likelihood, ensures optimal starting value for the EM algorithm. The use of the high number of maximum iterations and the small value of ε ensures that the fully iterated maximum likelihood estimator is obtained. This is an important condition for the use of this algorithm to bootstrap the number of components k.

4.6 Adjusting for Covariates

4.6.1 Generalized Linear Models

For the distributions considered in this monograph, adjusting for covariates leads to generalized linear models. This includes the normal, Poisson, negative binomial, and exponential distributions. Before covariate-adjusted finite mixture models are introduced, generalized linear models as formulated by Nelder and Wedderburn (1972) are briefly described. An overview of the theory and applications of generalized linear models may be found in the books by McCulloch and Searle (2001), McCullagh and Nelder (1989), Dobson (2008) and Aitkin et al. (2006). For generalized linear models it is assumed that observations y_i come from a distribution in the exponential family, that is,

$$f(y_i, \theta_i, \phi) = \exp\left(\frac{y_i\theta_i - b(\theta_i)}{a_i(\phi)} + c(y_i, \phi)\right), \tag{4.46}$$

where θ_i and ϕ are parameters and $a(\cdot), b(\cdot)$, and $c(\cdot)$ are specific and known functions. In all models considered here, $a_i(\phi)$ has the form

$$a_i(\phi) = \phi/p_i, \tag{4.47}$$

where p_i denotes a known *prior* weight; usually $p_i = 1$. Taking logs leads to the log likelihood function:

$$\log f(y_i, \theta_i, \phi) = \ell(\theta_i, \phi, y_i) = \frac{y_i\theta_i - b(\theta_i)}{a_i(\phi)} + c(y_i, \phi). \tag{4.48}$$

Using the results with regard to the expectation of the score (5.70) on page 138 leads to the following results for the expectation μ_i and the variance σ_i^2 of the random variable Y_i:

$$E\left(\frac{\partial \ell}{\partial \theta_i}\right) = E\left(\frac{y_i - b'(\theta)}{a_i(\phi)}\right) = 0. \tag{4.49}$$

Thus,

$$E(Y_i) = \mu_i = b'(\theta_i). \tag{4.50}$$

Likewise, using (5.71), we obtain

$$E\left(\frac{\partial^2 \ell}{\partial \theta_i^2}\right) + E\left(\frac{\partial \ell}{\partial \theta_i}\right)^2 = 0. \tag{4.51}$$

With $\mu_i = b'(\theta_i)$ the variance is given by

$$\text{var}(Y_i) = E\left[(y_i - b'(\theta_i))^2\right]. \tag{4.52}$$

Using the well-known formula

$$0 = -\frac{b''}{a_i(\phi)} + \frac{\text{var}(Y_i)}{a_i(\phi)^2}, \tag{4.53}$$

we obtain the variance as

$$\text{var}(Y_i) = -b''(\theta_i)a_i(\phi). \tag{4.54}$$

Here $b'(\cdot)$ and $b''(\cdot)$ denote the first and the second derivative of $b(\theta_i)$.

Example 4.5. Consider the Poisson density (3.1) on page 29. Substituting x with y and taking logs using the natural logarithm gives

$$\log f(y_i) = y_i \log \lambda_i - \lambda_i - \log(y_i!). \tag{4.55}$$

Looking at the coefficients of y_i, it is obvious that $\theta_i = \log \lambda_i$. Likewise, $c(y_i, \phi) = -\log(y_i!)$. Hence, $\lambda_i = e^{\theta_i}$ and as a result the second term can be written as $b(\theta_i) = e^{\theta_i}$. Finally, set the dispersion parameter $a(\phi) = \phi$ and $\phi = 1$. Thus, $E(Y) = b' = e^{\theta_i} = \lambda_i$ and $\text{var}(Y) = a_i(\phi)b''(\theta_i) = \lambda_i$.

Example 4.6. As another example consider the exponential distribution with $f(y) = \lambda e^{-\lambda y}$. Taking logs gives

$$\log f(y_i) = -y_i \lambda_i + \log \lambda_i. \tag{4.56}$$

Obviously $\theta_i = \lambda_i$ and $c(y_i, \phi) = 0$. Thus, the second term can be written as $b(\theta_i) = \log \theta_i$. Finally, set the dispersion parameter $a(\phi) = \phi$ and $\phi = 1$. As a result, $E(Y) = b'(\theta) = \frac{1}{\lambda_i}$ and $\text{var}(Y) = a_i(\phi)b''(\theta_i) = \frac{1}{\lambda_i^2}$.

The second part of the generalization of the linear model is that instead of modeling directly the mean a one-to-one continuous differentiable transformation of the mean $g(\mu_i)$ is introduced:

$$\eta_i = g(\mu_i). \tag{4.57}$$

The function $g(\cdot)$ is called the *link* function and introduces the transformed mean. The link function satisfies necessary constraints, such as $\mu > 0$ for Poisson-distributed count data. It is further assumed that the transformed mean follows a linear model, such that

$$\eta_i = x_i\beta. \tag{4.58}$$

The quantity η_i is the linear predictor, where $x_i = (x_{i1}, x_{i2}, \ldots, x_{im})$ is a row of the design matrix X and β is a vector of unknown regression coefficients. Since the link function is a one-to-one transformation, it can be inverted to obtain

$$\mu_i = g^{-1}(x_i\beta). \tag{4.59}$$

Example 4.7. For the Poisson distribution, the so-called canonical link function is the logarithm, since $\lambda_i = e^{x_i\beta}$.

Note that a generalized linear model consists of three ingredients. The first part involves a distribution from the exponential family, the second part is the linear predictor, and the final part is the link function. Since the link function is a strictly monotonic function, it can be inverted to map the linear predictor to the scale of the observations y_i. For the Poisson distribution this is achieved by exponentiating the linear predictor.

Maximum Likelihood Estimation for Generalized Linear Models

The standard approach to estimate the parameters of generalized linear models is via maximum likelihood. The log likelihood function is given by

$$\ell(\beta) = \sum_{i=1}^{n} \frac{y_i\theta_i - b(\theta)}{a_i(\phi)} + \sum_{i=1}^{n} c(y_i, \phi). \tag{4.60}$$

The likelihood equation when differentiating (4.60) with respect to β can be written as (McCullagh and Nelder 1989, pp. 40–43)

$$\frac{\partial \ell}{\partial \beta_j} = \sum_{i=1}^{n} w_i \frac{y_i - \mu_i}{a_i(\phi)} \frac{d\eta_i}{d\mu_i} x_{ij} = 0, \tag{4.61}$$

with weights w_i defined as

$$w_i = \tau_i / \left[b''(\theta_i) \left(\frac{d\eta_i}{d\mu_i} \right)^2 \right]. \tag{4.62}$$

Here $b''(\cdot)$ is the second derivative evaluated at θ and $a_i(\phi)$ takes the usual form: ϕ/τ_i, with weights τ_i. Usually (4.61) cannot be solved analytically, since it is non-linear in β; hence, an iterative algorithm is required. All generalized linear models can be fit using the same algorithm, namely, iterative weighted least squares.

Using starting values $\hat{\beta}$, the first step of the algorithm calculates the estimated linear predictor $\hat{\eta}_i = x_i\beta$. This is used to calculate the fitted values $\hat{\mu}_i = g^{-1}(\mu_i)$. On the basis of these quantities the so-called working dependent variable z_i is calculated

$$z_i = \hat{\eta}_i + (y_i - \hat{\mu}_i) \frac{d\eta_i}{d\mu_i}, \tag{4.63}$$

where the rightmost term is the derivative of the link function evaluated at the trial estimate. In the next step iterative weights are calculated according to (4.62). These weights w_i are inversely proportional to the variance of the working variate z_i based on the current parameter estimates and proportionality factor ϕ. Finally, a new estimate of β is obtained regressing the working dependent variable z_i on the predictors x_i using weights w_i, that is, in matrix notation

$$\hat{\beta} = (X^{\mathrm{T}}WX)^{-1}X^{\mathrm{T}}Wz, \tag{4.64}$$

where X is the design matrix and W is a diagonal matrix of weights with entries w_i defined in (4.62). Finally, z is a response vector with entries z_i defined in (4.63). This procedure is repeated until successive estimates change by less than a specified small amount, e.g., $\varepsilon = 0.00001$. These steps form the iterative weighted least squares algorithm for generalized linear models are summarized in Algorithm 4.6.1.

Step 0: Choose a vector of starting values $\hat{\beta}^{(0)}$ and calculate $\hat{\eta}$

Step 1: Calculate a working variate $z_i = \hat{\eta}_i + (y_i - \hat{\mu}_i)\frac{\mathrm{d}\eta_i}{\mathrm{d}\mu_i}$

Step 2: Calculate weights $w_i = \tau_i / \left[b''(\theta_i) \left(\frac{\mathrm{d}\eta_i}{\mathrm{d}\mu_i} \right)^2 \right]$

Step 3: Estimate $\hat{\beta}^{(l)} = (X^{\mathrm{T}}WX)^{-1}X^{\mathrm{T}}Wz$

Step 4: Calculate $\hat{\eta}$ based on $\hat{\beta}^{(l)}$ and go to step 1

Algorithm 4.6.1: Iterative weighted least squares algorithm for generalized linear models

Example 4.8. Consider a Poisson regression model with canonical link, that is, we model $\eta_i = \log(\lambda_i) = x_I\beta$. The derivative of the link function is given by $\frac{\mathrm{d}\eta_i}{\mathrm{d}\lambda_i} = \frac{1}{\lambda_i}$. Then the working variate is given by

$$z_i = \hat{\eta}_i + \frac{y_i - \hat{\lambda}_i}{\lambda_i}. \tag{4.65}$$

The iterative weight, with $\tau_i = 1$, is given by

$$w_i = 1 / \left[b''(\theta_i) \left(\frac{\mathrm{d}\eta_i}{\mathrm{d}\mu_i} \right)^2 \right]$$

$$= 1 / \left(\lambda_i \frac{1}{\lambda_i^2} \right) = \lambda_i. \tag{4.66}$$

Again, the weights are inversely proportional to the variance of the working variate.

4.6.2 The EM Algorithm for Covariate-Adjusted Mixture Models

There is a growing body of literature on covariate-adjusted finite mixture models. See, for example, McLachlan and Peel (2000), Wedel (2002), Viele and Tong (2002), Ng and McLachlan (2003), Xiang et al. (2005), or Frühwirth-Schnatter (2006). The starting point of the covariate-adjusted mixture model is the definition of the mixture density of the response variable Y_i belonging to the exponential family. In this case the mixture density with k components is defined as

$$f(y_i, P) = \sum_{j=1}^{k} p_j f(y_i, \theta_{ij}, \phi_j) \quad j = 1, \ldots, k, \tag{4.67}$$

where the log density for the jth component is given by

$$\log f(y_i, \theta_{ij}) = \frac{y_i \theta_{ij} - b(\theta_{ij})}{a_i(\phi_j)} + c(y_i, \phi_{ij}). \tag{4.68}$$

Typically, for each mixture component the same density is assumed and thus for the jth component μ_{ij} denotes the mean of Y_i, $g(\cdot)$ denotes the link function, and $\eta_j = g(\mu_{ij}) = x_i^T \beta_j$ denotes the linear predictor. Thus, each component is described by a generalized linear model with a different linear predictor, but the same error distribution and the same link function. The semiparametric mixing distribution may now be written as in (3.13) on page 33. This leads to

$$P \equiv \begin{bmatrix} \lambda_1 & \cdots & \lambda_k \\ p_1 & \cdots & p_k \end{bmatrix}. \tag{4.69}$$

Now the parameters $\lambda_1, \ldots, \lambda_k$ are no longer scalar quantities, but vectors, e.g.,

$$\lambda_1 = (\beta_{01}, \beta_{11}, \ldots, \beta_{m1}), \tag{4.70}$$

where m denotes the number of covariates in the model. As before p_j, $j = 1, \ldots, k$ denotes the mixing weights. Since the error distribution and the link function are assumed to be identical for each component, the componentwise vectors of regression coefficients are the systematic part of the model.

Example 4.9. A covariate-adjusted finite mixture model based on the Poisson distribution may be written as

$$f(y_i, P) = \sum_{j=1}^{k} p_j f(y_i, \lambda_j), \ \lambda_j = \exp(x_i \lambda_j) \quad j = 1, \ldots, k. \tag{4.71}$$

Here, a logarithmic link is assumed and λ_j denotes the vector of regression coefficients of the jth component.

The EM Algorithm

The EM algorithm for covariate-adjusted finite mixture models is again based on the complete data likelihood and in this case is given by

$$\log L_c(P) = \sum_{i=1}^{n}\sum_{j=1}^{k} z_{ij}\log p_i + \sum_{i=1}^{n}\sum_{j=1}^{k} z_{ij}\log f(y_i,\theta_{ij},\phi_j). \qquad (4.72)$$

As before the E-step of the EM algorithm involves replacing the unobserved indicator variables z_{ij} with their expected values given the data $(y_1,\ldots,y_n)$. Thus, the E-step denotes the posterior probability of the ith observation belonging to the jth component and is given by

$$e_{ij} = \frac{p_j f(y_i,\theta_{ij},\phi_j)}{\sum_l p_l f(y_i,\theta_{il},\phi_l)}. \qquad (4.73)$$

The M-step involves maximization of the current expected complete data likelihood. For the mixing weights this is again given by the simple formula

$$p_j^{\text{new}} = \frac{\sum_i e_{ij}}{n} = \sum_i \frac{p_j f(y_i,\theta_{ij},\phi_j)}{\sum_l p_l f(y_i,\theta_{il},\phi_l)}\Big/n. \qquad (4.74)$$

Concerning the computation of the component parameters β_j they are estimated by finding the maximum likelihood estimate for the second sum of the expected complete data likelihood. This implies that the solution of the following equation needs to be obtained:

$$\sum_{i=1}^{n}\sum_{j=1}^{k} e_{ij}\frac{\partial}{\partial \beta}\log f(y_i,\theta_{ij},\phi_j) = 0. \qquad (4.75)$$

It follows from Sect. 4.6.1 on homogenous generalized linear models that (4.75) can be written as

$$\sum_{i=1}^{n}\sum_{j=1}^{k} e_{ij}w_i\frac{y_i-\mu_{ij}}{a_i(\phi_j)}\frac{d\eta_i}{d\mu_i}x_i = 0. \qquad (4.76)$$

Comparing (4.76) with (4.60) reveals that the former has the same form as a homogeneous generalized linear model with component-specific prior weights $\tau_{ij} = e_{ij}$. Note that for a full random effects model, i.e., if the parameter vectors β_j have no elements in common for each component, new estimates of β^{l+1} may be fit componentwise. If there are some common elements, the parameters β_j may be estimated using standard software packages for generalized linear models such as R or SAS.

This is achieved by expanding the response vector to have length $n \times k$. That is, for a mixture of generalized linear models with $k = 2$ components, the new response vector $\tilde{y}$ would have $n \times k$ elements. Likewise, the design matrix needs to be augmented as well. Usually a design matrix with n observations and m covariates would have dimension $n \times m$. Now for each covariate (including the intercept)

Table 4.2 Response vector $\tilde{y}$ and design matrix $\tilde{X}$ for the covariate-adjusted mixture model of the Ames test data

$\tilde{y}$	β_{01}	β_{02}	β_{03}	Dose	$\log(0.3 + \text{dose})$
11	1	0	0	0	-1.204
11	0	1	0	0	-1.204
11	0	0	1	0	-1.204
...	...	...	...	...	...
...	...	...	...	...	...
789	1	0	0	10	2.332
789	0	1	0	10	2.332
789	0	0	1	10	2.332

which will have random effects, the augmented design matrix $\tilde{X}$ needs to have k additional columns. Additionally, for each k, the number of rows of the augmented design matrix needs to be the same as for the augmented response vector.

Consider, for example, the design matrix for the finite mixture model in Sect. 3.5.3. The data set has $n = 100$ observations and uses the covariates dose and $\log(0.3 + \text{dose})$. The final mixture model has three components with different intercepts and common slopes. Thus, the response vector has length 100×3. The design matrix has $100 \times 3 = 300$ rows and $k + 2 = 5$ columns. The elements of the design matrix $\tilde{X}$ and the augmented response vector $\tilde{y}$ are shown in Table 4.2. On the basis of this design matrix with vectorized weights e_{ij} the parameter estimates β_j^{l+1} may be estimated using standard software. Thus, the EM algorithm for covariate-adjusted mixture models implies performing first the necessary data augmentation, and then based on starting values for p_j and β_j the computation of posterior probabilities e_{ij}. This is the E-step. In the M-step new mixing weights p_j and regression coefficients β_j are computed. This is summarized in Algorithm 4.6.2.

Step 0: Let P be any vector of starting values
Step 1. Compute the E-step according to (4.73)
Step 2: Compute the M-step according to (4.74) and (4.6.1), leading to $P^{(l)}$ and $\beta^{(l)}$
Step 3: Let $P = P^{(l)}$ and go to step 1

Algorithm 4.6.2: EM algorithm for covariate-adjusted mixture models

---

4.6.3 Computation: Vitamin A Supplementation Revisited

Covariate-adjusted finite mixture models can be fit with the function *covmix* of the R package CAMAN. To demonstrate its use we continue with our example of vitamin A supplementation and childhood mortality.

As an alternative to a "standard" meta-analysis we apply a covariate-adjusted finite mixture model to the data. Table 4.3 shows the data prepared for a Poisson

Table 4.3 Vitamin A supplementation: data prepared for Poisson regression. 0 indicates the control group and 1 denotes the vitamin A group

Location	Observation time	Cases	At risk	Treatment	Person time
Sarlahi (Nepal)	12	152	14,487	1	173,844
	12	210	14,143	0	169,716
Northern Sudan	18	123	14,446	1	260,028
	18	117	14,294	0	257,292
Tamil Nadu (India)	12	37	7,764	1	93,168
	12	80	7,655	0	91,860
Aceh (Indonesia)	12	101	12,991	1	155,892
	12	130	12,209	0	146,508
Hyderabad (India)	12	39	7,691	1	92,292
	12	41	8,084	0	97,008
Jumla (Nepal)	5	138	3,786	1	18,930
	5	167	3,411	0	17,055
Java (Indonesia)	12	186	5,775	1	69,300
	12	250	5,445	0	65,340
Mumbai (India)	42	7	1,784	1	74,928
	42	32	1,664	0	69,888

regression model. Here the covariate treatment uses value 0 for the control and value 1 for the supplementation group. The analysis starts with a Poisson regression model using treatment as a covariate and person time (observation time × population at risk) as an offset. The corresponding call to the standard R function *glm* is as follows:

```
> library(CAMAN)
> data(vitamin)
> m0<-glm(cases~treatment,offset=log(py),family =
poisson(),data=vitamin)
```

This leads to the result

```
> m0


Coefficients:
(Intercept)        treatment
    -6.7919          -0.2969


Degrees of Freedom: 15 Total (i.e., Null);
14 Residual Null Deviance: 1683
Residual Deviance: 1644    AIC: 1748
```

It is of note that we find a protective effect of vitamin A supplementation on childhood mortality In the next step a covariate-adjusted mixture model is fit to the data.

We try a model with random intercepts and random slopes for treatment and $k = 3$ components. This is achieved with the call

```
> m3 <- mixcov(dep="cases", fixed=c("1"),
  random=c("treatment"),pop.at.risk=vitamin$py,
  family="poisson",data=vitamin, k=3)
```

In contrast to the function *glm*, the logarithm of person time is calculated within the function *mixcov*.

The result is given by

```
> m3

Data consist of 16 observations (rows).

mixing weights:
  comp. 1    comp. 2    comp. 3
0.4375004 0.3124996 0.2500000

 Coefficients :
 Z1              Z2              Z3
-7.711          -6.879          -5.286

Z1:treatment Z2:treatment Z3:treatment
 -0.124         -0.294         -0.321

Log-Likelihood: -167.3646     BIC: 356.91
```

The BIC of model *m1* is 1,748.773, whereas the current model has a BIC of 356.91, which is considerably better. Note that besides treatment heterogeneity there is, according to varying intercepts, also baseline heterogeneity present. This information is not available in a "standard" meta-analysis.

4.6.4 An Extension of the EM Algorithm with Gradient Update for Covariate-Adjusted Mixture Models

The EM algorithm (Sect. 4.6.2) is known to converge often only to a local maximum. As a result, this section introduces an extension of the EM algorithm which incorporates information from the gradient as outlined in Sect. 4.4.6 for finite mixture models.

The crucial part in extending Algorithm 4.4.3 for covariate-adjusted finite mixture models is step 3 where finding λ_{max} is required to maximize the gradient $d(\lambda_j, \hat{P}_{EM})$. This was discussed by Seidel et al. (2006) for mixtures of exponentials. Finding λ_{max} implies finding the maximum of a potentially high dimensional function in the case of covariate-adjusted mixture models.

For that reason the use of simulated annealing, as a stochastic optimization algorithm, is introduced to find the maximum of the gradient function. The idea of simulated annealing comes from statistical mechanics. Here the behavior of a system of particles undergoing a change in temperature is of interest. At high temperatures the molecules of a liquid move freely with respect to one another. If the liquid is cooled slowly, thermal mobility is lost. For slowly cooled systems nature finds a state of minimum energy where the atoms line themselves up and form a pure crystal. This crystal is the state of minimum energy (Press et al. 2007). Kirkpatrick et al. (1983) introduced simulated annealing as a general optimization technique. Robert and Casella (2004) translated these ideas into statistical terms.

The basic idea in statistical terms is that a change in *temperature* T allows for faster moves on the surface of the function f to be maximized. The negative of this function is called *energy*. As a result, rescaling the temperature T avoids the trapping in local maxima. Given a temperature $T > 0$, a potentially vector valued sample $\lambda_1, \lambda_2, \ldots$ is generated from the distribution

$$\pi(\lambda) \propto \exp(f(\lambda)/T).$$

This distribution can be used to find the maximum of $f(\lambda)$. As T decreases towards zero, the values simulated from this distribution become concentrated in a narrower neighborhood of the maxima of $f(\lambda)$. This becomes clearer when the simulation method proposed by Metropolis et al. (1953) is used. Starting from λ_0, a value ξ is generated from a uniform distribution in the neighborhood $\upsilon(\lambda_0)$ and the new value λ is generated as follows:

$$\lambda_1 = \begin{cases} \xi, & \text{with probability } \pi = \exp(\Delta f/T) \wedge 1, \\ \lambda_0, & \text{with probability } 1 - \pi, \end{cases} \tag{4.77}$$

where $\Delta f = f(\xi) - f(\lambda_0)$. Thus, if $f(\xi) > f(\lambda_0)$, ξ is accepted with probability 1 and λ_0 is changed into ξ. Otherwise if $f(\xi) < f(\lambda_0)$, ξ may still be accepted with probability $\pi \neq 0$ and λ_0 is changed into ξ. This property allows the algorithm to escape a local maximum with a probability which depends on the temperature T. This idea leads to the general simulated annealing Algorithm 4.6.3.

Step 1: Simulate ξ from a distribution with density $g(|\xi - \theta_0|)$
Step 2: Accept λ_{i+1} with probability $\pi = \exp(f(\Delta f/T) \wedge 1$ and take $\lambda_{i+1} = \lambda_i$ otherwise
Step 3: Update T_i to T_{i+1}

Algorithm 4.6.3: Simulated annealing

To apply this algorithm to find the maximum of the potential multidimensional gradient function, the result of the first step of Algorithm 4.6.2 is used. That is, the solution λ_{EM} of the EM algorithm for covariate-adjusted mixture models provides starting values for simulated annealing. Simulate now ξ in the neighborhood of λ_{EM}. This implies using the result of the EM iterations and finding a new random configuration of λ_{EM}. If this configuration leads to a larger value of the gradient, then this configuration is accepted. Otherwise, choose a uniform random number u on the interval $[0, 1]$. If

$$u < \exp\left(\frac{D(\xi, P) - D(\lambda.P)}{T}\right),\tag{4.78}$$

then the new configuration is accepted as well; otherwise the current configuration remains unchanged. Then in the next step the temperature is decreased. This algorithm is summarized in Algorithm 4.6.4.

Step 1: Choose an initial configuration λ_{EM} given by the result of the EM algorithm, initial and final temperatures T_0 and T_f

Step 2: Simulate a new configuration ξ in the neighborhood of λ_i based on a uniform distribution $U(-r, r)$

Step 3: If $D(\xi, P) > D(\lambda, P)$, then $\lambda_{i+1} = \xi$.
Otherwise choose random u in the range $(0, 1)$.
If $u < \exp\left(\frac{D(\xi, P) - D(\lambda.P)}{T}\right)$, then $\lambda_{i+1} = \xi$, otherwise $\lambda_{i+1} = \lambda_i$

Step 4: Update T_i to T_{i+1} and go to step 2

Algorithm 4.6.4: Simulated annealing step of the hybrid EM gradient update algorithm

4.7 Case Study: EM Algorithm with Gradient Update for Nonlinear Finite Mixture Models

4.7.1 Introduction

Population pharmacokinetic analysis is an important task in drug development. This approach was introduced in Sect. 2.3. One of the most crucial parts is the choice of the distribution for the random effects. The most common choice is to assume a normal distribution for the random effects (Davidian and Giltinan 1995). Assuming a normal distribution has the disadvantage that the integrand inside the likelihood function has no closed-form solution. Thus, it has to be approximated, e.g., by a Taylor series expansion, Gaussian quadrature, or Monte Carlo integration (Pinheiro and Bates 1995). Alternatively a full Bayesian approach using Monte Carlo Markov chain methods can be applied.

Another approach is to assume a discrete distribution for the random effects, i.e., a finite mixture model. This idea was pioneered by Mallet (1986). The algorithm developed by Mallet fits random effects for all coefficients of the model. Hence, here we develop a variant of the EM algorithm which allows both fixed and random effects. The EM algorithm converges to a local maximum of the likelihood function (Dempster et al. 1977) where the particular solution is determined by the starting values. Thus, we apply the hybrid EM algorithm with gradient update described in the previous section.

4.7.2 Example: Dipyrone Pharmacokinetics

Dipyrone is an analgesic, antipyretic, and anti-inflammatory drug still widely used in many countries. It is also known under the names metamizole, noramidopyrine, methampyrone, and sulpyrine, as well as brand names Analgin, Novalgin, Baralgan, and Ultragin.

Although Dipyrone is recognized as an effective analgesic, anti-inflammatory, and antipyretic, its in humans is controversial. Since the 1930s it has been known that Dipyrone can cause agranulocytosis (severe reduction in the number of white blood cells). Prior to the connection with Dipyrone, this adverse drug reaction had already been observed with another drug, amidopyrine, which has a similar chemical structure. Owing to the link with agranulocytosis, Dipyrone has been banned in many countries (including the USA, the UK, and Sweden).

However, there is general disagreement about the increase in risk of agranulo-cytosis associated with Dipyrone use. A large case-control study was conducted in Europe and Israel, the so-called Agranulocytosis and Aplastic Anaemia (IAAA) study. The results, published in 1986, reported an estimate of the risk at an accept-ably low level of 1.1 cases per million users (IAAAS 1986). A more recent analysis of Dipyrone-related agranulocytosis in Sweden estimated the risk to be much higher, one case per 1,439 users (Hedenmalm and Spigset 2002).

Its pharmacokinetics are characterized by rapid hydrolysis to the active moiety, 4-methylaminoantipyrine (MAA), which has 85% bioavailability after oral admin-istration in tablet form. MAA is further metabolized to 4-formylaminoantipyrine, which is an end metabolite, and to 4-aminoantipyrine, which is further acetylated to 4-acetylaminoantipyrine by the polymorphic N-acetyltransferase. The analgesic effect of Dipyrone was found to correlate mainly to the time course of MAA (Levy et al. 1995).

Our analysis deals with an experimental data set that was compiled in the course of a phase I clinical trial conducted by Flusser et al. (1988). This data set ex-hibits the high design restrictions associated with experimental data, with 12 healthy volunteers each being administered the same dose orally and measurements being recorded at a number of predetermined time points.

For an initial graphical analysis of the data, plots of MAA concentration versus time are constructed. The concentration–time curves for each of the 12 subjects are plotted in Fig. 4.15.

The individual plots indicate that there is substantial interindividual variability in the disposition of Dipyrone and an analysis taking heterogeneity between individu-als into account seems appropriate.

4.7.3 First-Order Compartment Models

Because Dipyrone was administered orally, we assume a first-order absorption rate as in Fig. 2.5. The simplest model we can try is the one-compartment model with

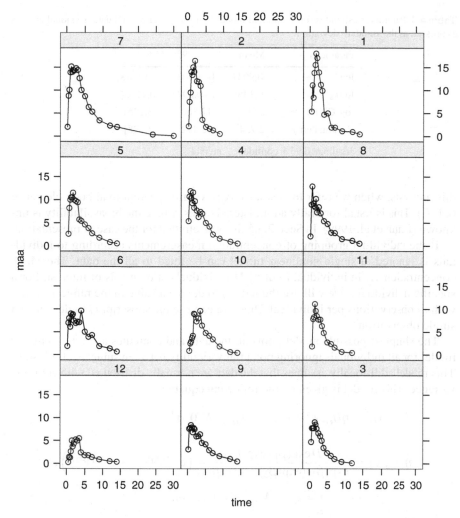

Fig. 4.15 Individual concentration–time curves for the metabolite 4-methylaminoantipyrine (*MAA*) in 12 healthy volunteers after oral administration of a single dose of Dipyrone

first-order absorption rate to describe the concentration $c(t)$ at time t (4.79). In this model k_a and k_e represent the constants of absorption and elimination , respectively, whereas Cl denotes the clearance (the amount of drug cleared from the body per unit time):

$$c(t) = \frac{Dk_a k_e}{\text{Cl}(k_a - k_e)}(e^{-k_e t} - e^{-k_a t}), \tag{4.79}$$

where D denotes the dose given. For the model to be meaningful all parameters need to be positive. As a result, we use the following parameterization proposed by Pinheiro and Bates (2000): $\beta_1 = \log k_e$, $\beta_2 = \log k_a$, and $\beta_3 = \log(\text{Cl}/F)$. Throughout

Table 4.4 Parameter estimates for the pooled model fit to the experimental data. Residual error is expressed as the standard deviation

Parameter	Mean	95% CI[a]	
$\log k_e$	−0.9941	[−1.503	−0.4848]
$\log k_a$	−0.1389	[−0.692	0.4145]
$\log(\text{Cl}/F)$	2.997	[2.860	3.135]
Residual error	2.734	[2.492	3.028]

[a]Estimated 95% confidence interval

this analysis, when we refer to clearance (Cl) we use apparent total body clearance (Cl/F). This is usual for orally administered doses, where the bioavailability is unknown (Lunn et al. 1999). In Sect. 2.3.5 this was omitted for the ease of presentation.

If the individual grouping of concentration measurements according to individuals is ignored, a single nonlinear model can be fitted to all the data. The MAA concentration y_{ij} in individual i out of M individuals at time t_j is of interest. For a specific individual i, we will use the letter j to denote a value in the range $1, \ldots, n_i$, with n_i observations per individual Thus, we can use the subscript ij to designate a single observation.

The simplest possible model pools all the data and computes a single nonlinear model for all individuals ignoring potential variability between subjects (Table 4.4). This model additionally assumes that the data are normally distributed with common variance. This model is given by the following equation:

$$y_{ij} = \eta(t_{ij}, \lambda) + \varepsilon_{ij}, \qquad \varepsilon_{ij} \sim N(0, \sigma^2)$$

$$\eta(t_{ij}, \lambda) = \frac{D \exp(\beta_1) \exp(\beta_2)}{\exp(\beta_3)(\exp(\beta_2) - \exp(\beta_1))} \left(e^{-\exp(\beta_1)t_j} - e^{-\exp(\beta_2)t} \right),$$

$$i = 1, \ldots, M, \quad j = 1, \ldots, n_i.$$

The parameter vector $\lambda = (\beta_1, \beta_2, \beta_3)$ needs to be estimated from the data. This can be done using maximum likelihood or nonlinear least squares (Bates and Watts 1988).

This model was fit using maximum likelihood with corresponding log likelihood of −448.07. However, looking at Fig. 4.16, we can see that for some individuals the residuals are mostly positive, while for others they are mostly negative. This indicates heterogeneity between individuals. Thus, a common model for all individuals doe not seem to be appropriate.

If there are sufficient data, one can attempt to fit a nonlinear model to the concentration–time curve of each individual. Using the one-compartment model, we attempt to fit the data for each of M individuals separately. Thus, we can consider M separate nonlinear regression problems, the ith model being expressed by

Fig. 4.16 Boxplots of residuals grouped by subject for the pooled model

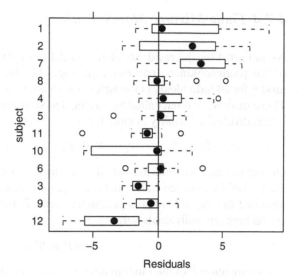

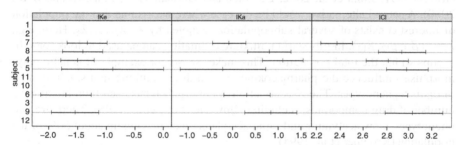

Fig. 4.17 Ninety-five percent confidence intervals for the estimates of the three pharmacokinetic parameters according to a one-compartment model fit to the data of each subject separately

$$y_{ij} = \eta(t_{ij}, \lambda_i) + \varepsilon_{ij}, \quad i = 1, \ldots, M, \ j = 1, \ldots, n_i, \ \varepsilon_i \sim N(0, \sigma^2). \qquad (4.80)$$

Here y_{ij} denotes the measured concentration on the jth observation of individual i with n_i observations. The combined statistical parameters are $\lambda_i = (\beta_{1i}, \beta_{2i}, \beta_{3i}, \ i = 1, \ldots, M)$.

For six out of the 12 subjects in the experimental data set, the nonlinear least-squares algorithm fails. Apparently, the data exhibit complex characteristics that make fitting a simple one-compartment model difficult.

Confidence intervals for the estimates of the three pharmacokinetic parameters in each individual are a useful means of assessing whether the parameters differ significantly from one individual to another (see Fig. 4.17). Judging from this Fig. 4.17, we could say that clearance and absorption rate show significant variability, while the elimination rate does vary very substantially from one individual to another.

4.7.4 Finite Mixture Model Analysis

As indicated by the residuals of the model in (4.80) and the confidence intervals of the pharmacokinetic parameters in Fig. 4.17, the assumption of a homogenous model for all individuals is too strict. This leads to nonlinear mixed effects models. These models are often called hierarchical models. On the first level of the hierarchy intraindividual variability is modeled as

$$y_{ij} = \eta(t_{ij}, \lambda_i) + \varepsilon_{ij}, \qquad \varepsilon_{ij} \sim N(0, \sigma^2), \quad i = 1, \ldots, M, \quad j = 1, \ldots, n_i. \quad (4.81)$$

On the second level interindividual variability is modeled. Here, it is assumed that the variability between individuals can again be described by a distribution P. It is assumed that the individual's parameter vector λ_i follows a distribution with mean μ and between-individuals variance Ψ:

$$\lambda_i \sim P(\mu, \Psi). \qquad (4.82)$$

The distribution P of the random effects is often assumed to be normal (Sheiner and Grasela 1991; Lunn et al. 2002; Davidian and Giltinan 1995; Pinheiro and Bates 2000). A natural alternative would be the case where we assume that the population of interest consists of several subpopulations denoted by $\lambda_1, \lambda_2, \ldots, \lambda_k$. Here, e.g., $\lambda_1 = (\beta_{11}, \beta_{12}, \beta_{13})$. In this setting, mixture estimation can be used to look for subgroups within the total population. This makes sense, for example, if genetic polymorphisms influence the pharmacokinetics of a drug, resulting in a small number of distinct phenotypes. The N-acetylation polymorphism has been found to affect a number of drug compounds, including Dipyrone (Levy et al. 1995). There are two phenotypes, slow acetylator and rapid acetylator, each making up about 50% of the population (Kroemer et al. 1994).

In a mixture model, in contrast to the homogenous case we have the same type of density for each subpopulation but a different parameter vector λ_j in subpopulation j. In our population $Y_1, Y_2, \ldots, Y_M$ it is not observed to which subpopulation the ith individual with its measurements $y_i = y_{i1}, \ldots, y_{in_i}$ belongs. Therefore, this phenomenon is called *unobserved heterogeneity*. If we take this into account, the conditional distribution is given by

$$y_i \sim p_1 f(y_i, \lambda_1) + \cdots + p_k f(y_i, \lambda_k) \quad k \quad \text{components}$$

$$f(y_i, \lambda_j) = \prod_l^{n_i} N(y_{il}, \eta(t_{il}, \lambda_j), \sigma) \quad n_i \quad \text{observations.}$$

Assuming conditional independence for each individual, the density $f(\cdot)$ is given by the product of the normal densities of this individual. Conditional independence means that while the observations from a single individual are not independent of one another, observations from different individuals are independent and furthermore, conditional on the random effects b_i, all observations are independent. We shall use this assumption in the next section to develop an expression for the likelihood of this model.

Each mixture component is described by a separate nonlinear regression model with parameter vector λ_j. The discrete finite random parameter P is given by

Table 4.5 Parameter estimates for the three component mixture model fit to the experimental data. Residual error is expressed as the standard deviation

Parameter	Group 1 (0.6%)	Group 2 (16.38%)	Group 3 (83.02%)
$\log k_e$	7.894	−0.9783	−1.0219
$\log k_a$	−2.794	−0.9912	0.0125
$\log(Cl/F)$	−3.836	−3.7146	−3.968
Residual error		5.1766	

$$P = \begin{bmatrix} \lambda_1 \ldots \lambda_k \\ p_1 \ldots p_k \end{bmatrix},$$

with $\lambda_j = (\beta_{j1}, \ldots, \beta_{jm})^T$, m parameters, and $j = 1, \ldots, k$ components.

Coefficients λ_j, mixing weights p_j, and the number of components k must be estimated from the data, e.g., using maximum likelihood using the EM algorithm. Alternatively a variant of the VDM algorithm might be used (Lai and Shih 2003). Here we start with the basic EM algorithm. The result is shown in Table 4.5 and is truly disappointing. The log likelihood is −466.948, which is much worse than the fit of the simple pooled model with a log likelihood of −448.07. Likewise, the residual standard error is larger than that estimated by the pooled model.

Possible reasons for this result lie in the fact that the likelihood for mixtures has many local maxima. Also the results of the EM algorithm depend on starting values as noted by Seidel et al. (2000b) and Seidel and Sevcikova (2004). Thus, here the EM algorithm with gradient update for mixture models with covariates as described in Sect. 4.6.4 is applied to the data.

Figure 4.18 shows that indeed using the hybrid EM algorithm the local maximum can be left and the potential global maximum is reached. Likewise, looking at the

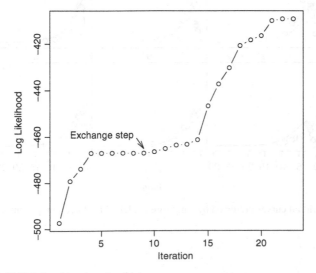

Fig. 4.18 Hybrid EM algorithm iteration history

Table 4.6 Parameter estimates for the three component mixture model fit to the experimental data. Residual error is expressed as the standard deviation

Parameter	Group 1 (25%)	Group 2 (16.6%)	Group 3 (58.4%)
$\log k_e$	−0.5590	−0.9551	−1.305
$\log k_a$	−0.5084	−1.032	0.4078
$\log(Cl/F)$	2.705	3.200	3.014
Residual error		1.668	

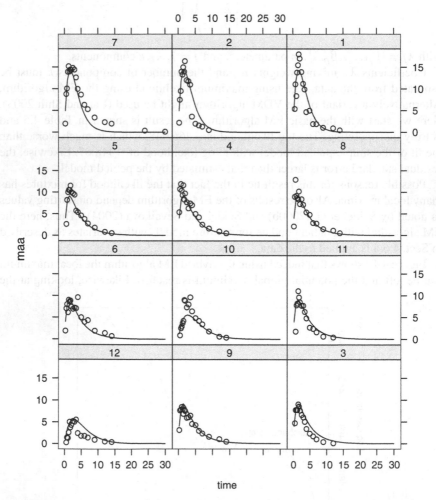

Fig. 4.19 Individual curves predicted by a mixture model with a three-component fit to the experimental data

corresponding log likelihoods, a much better fit is obvious. The log likelihood of the current model is -409.215. The previous log likelihood of the solution provided by the EM algorithm was -448.07. The results of this model are shown in Table 4.6.

This model indicates variability in absorption, clearance, and elimination. Looking at Fig. 4.19, the fit of this model is much better than that of the pooled model, but there seems to be room for improvement. Likewise, to fit this model, a large number of parameters have to be estimated, that is, a total of 11. However, this result is a good starting point for other population pharmacokinetic analyses since this result can be used as a starting value for sparse data. Work is in progress to analyze data from a study performed by Levy et al. (2007) using a finite mixture model. Levy et al. used a model which relies on a normal distribution for the random effects. A recent simulation study (Bustad et al. 2006) has shown that finite mixture models are often superior with regard to performance and thus this reanalysis is in progress.

Chapter 5
Disease Mapping and Cluster Investigations

5.1 Introduction

Geographic epidemiology has become a popular tool in epidemiology and public health. A general overview of applications and methods of spatial or geographic epidemiology may be found in the books by Lawson et al. (1999) and Elliott et al. (2000) or in the *Handbook of Epidemiology*, where Bithell (2007) provides an introduction to the field. An overview on advanced statistical methods for spatial epidemiology is given in the monograph by Lawson (2006).

Applications

The use of geographic epidemiology includes the construction of cancer atlases which are often applied to generate hypotheses about the causes of disease. One such example is the second edition of the German cancer atlas (Becker et al. 1984). Maps of stomach cancer revealed higher rates in northeast Bavaria, which led to subsequent analytic studies identifying risk factors for stomach cancer in that area. Another application is given in health care evaluation. One example is the access to expert psychiatric services in the city of Hamburg (Maylath et al. 2000a,b). These studies, based on routine data, identified factors which influence access to specialist care. One of these factors is the social status of patients. Other applications deal with the regional distribution of "avoidable deaths" caused by potentially fatal diseases which can be cured by modern medical treatment. Holland (1993) collected data on such deaths throughout the European Community and presented it in the form of maps and tables. Schlattmann (2000) investigated the regional distribution of breast cancer mortality in women in Germany 1995 and identified differences in mortality between rural and urban areas and the western and eastern parts of Germany.

A more prominent application is so-called *cluster* investigations. Frequently, there is public concern about putative disease clusters around a presumed hazardous institution. Famous examples are given by the leukemia cluster around Sellafield in the UK or the cluster of childhood leukemia around the nuclear power plant at

Krümmel in Germany. There is an ongoing debate whether these clusters can be linked to a single exposure such as a nuclear power plant (Alexander et al. 1998; Bellec et al. 2006; Bithell 2001). Recently, this discussion was fueled by new findings of the German childhood cancer registry (Kaatsch et al. 2008; Spix et al. 2008). The researchers performed a case-control study with population-based matched controls (1:3) which were selected from the corresponding registrar's office. Residential proximity to the nearest nuclear power plant was determined for each subject individually with a precision of about 25 m. The study focused on leukemia and mainly on cases in the inner 5-km zone around the plants. A categorical analysis showed a statistically significant odds ratio of 2.19 (lower 95% confidence level 1.51) for residential proximity within 5 km compared with residence outside this area.

The cause of (childhood) leukemia is largely unknown. In this framework several hypotheses are under discussion. One of these is the Gardner hypothesis (Gardner et al. 1990) suggesting that an excess of childhood leukemia near a nuclear installation is caused by parental exposure to ionizing radiation. Besides the environmental hypothesis, an infectious cause is discussed as well, which is the so-called 'Kinlen' hypothesis (Kinlen 1988, 1997). This hypotheses states that population mixing and infection are a possible explanation for the clusters of childhood acute leukemia around nuclear processing plants. More precisely Kinlen's hypothesis implies that population groups who were relatively isolated in the past but have recently received a large influx of newcomers may experience an increase in the incidence of childhood leukemia, because of changes in herd immunity. Another hypothesis in this context is Greaves's hypothesis. Greaves formulated the hypothesis that delayed exposure to common infections leads to an increased risk of childhood leukemia, especially common pre-B acute lymphoblastic leukemia (ALL). Childhood ALL is considered to be a rare response to common infections (Greaves 1988, 1997; Greaves and Alexander 1993). The pathogenesis of leukemia is believed to occur in two phases. The first genetic event is considered to take place during the expansion of B-cell precursors in pregnancy. The second genetic event is thought to occur in the same mutant clone, following an immune stress, such as a common infection. The delayed exposure to infection is considered to increase the number of target cells, with the "first hit" present at older ages. On the basis of this hypothesis, a child isolated from infectious agents at the beginning of his/her life would have a higher risk of acquiring ALL, while a high birth order value, early common infections, and early day care would be protective factors.

However, when performing an investigation of a presumed cluster the question arises of how to define a cluster. A working definition of a cluster is given by Last (2000) in *A Dictionary of Epidemiology*:

Definition 5.1. 'Cluster: Aggregation of relatively uncommon events or diseases in space and/or time in amounts that are believed or perceived to be greater than could be expected by chance.'

Unfortunately, this definition does not provide a quantifiable and testable hypothesis. Thus, in analyzing putative clusters of disease, one may distinguish two main strategies. Besag and Newell (1991) described tests of clustering either as general or focused. Investigations that seek to address "general clustering" determine whether or not cases are clustered anywhere in the study area, without a prior assumption about the location of a potential cluster. In contrast, tests addressing "focused" clustering assess whether cases are clustered around a prespecified source of hazard, which is frequently called a focus. When dealing with focused investigations, the "Texas sharp shooter phenomenon" frequently occurs. It states that the target is defined after firing and thus hit perfectly. Thus, focused analyses may be biased by selecting the study area and the way exposure is operationalized. Therefore, from the author's point of view the analysis of "general clustering" should be a starting point of any cluster investigation.

5.2 Investigation of General Clustering

There has been debate in the media about whether there is excess childhood leukemia in the vicinity of the nuclear power plant at Rossendorf close to Dresden in the southeast of the former East Germany. The area is shown in Fig. 5.1. The data were analyzed by Böhning and Schlattmann (1999)[1] and the results are presented in the following section together with a more detailed description of empirical Bayes methods.

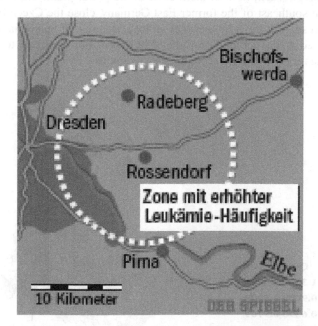

Fig. 5.1 Suspected childhood leukemia cluster in the area of Dresden as published in *Der Spiegel* (1996)

---

[1] The use of part of the material in this book is kindly permitted by John Wiley & Sons.

As already mentioned, the analysis of this potential focus is based on an analysis of generalized clustering to avoid a selection bias. In the following, the investigation of general clustering is based on disease mapping methods. Traditional approaches would include the construction of percentile or probability maps. In a first step the construction of disease maps requires the choice of an epidemiologic measure which shall be presented on a map. Frequently the standardized mortality ratio (SMR) of the individual region given by $\text{SMR}_i = \frac{o_i}{E_i}$ is used. Here, o_i denotes the number of observed cases, while E_i denotes the expected cases based on an internal standard, i.e., the age-specific rates of the total region.

5.2.1 Traditional Approaches

In our first example we present data from the former East Germany within the time period from 1980 to 1989. The data are taken from the cancer atlas of the former East Germany (Möhner et al. 1994). Traditional approaches of categorization are based on the percentiles of the SMR distribution. Most cancer atlases use this approach commonly based on quartiles, quintiles, or sextiles. The map shown in Fig. 5.2 presents the regional distribution of childhood leukemia in the former East Germany. According to this percentile map there is an increased risk in the districts of Sebnitz and Dresden, both of them close to the power plant. These districts are located in the southeast of the former East Germany, close the Czech border. This map seems to support the hypothesis of an increased risk of leukemia in that area. But maps based on the percentiles of the SMR distribution are likely to reflect only random fluctuations in the corresponding small counts.

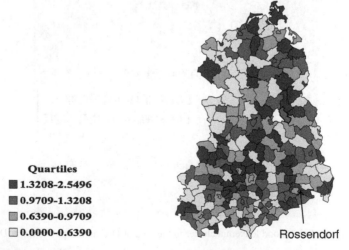

Quartiles
- ■ 1.3208–2.5496
- ■ 0.9709–1.3208
- ▨ 0.6390–0.9709
- ☐ 0.0000–0.6390

Rossendorf

Fig. 5.2 Childhood leukemia in the former East Germany from 1980 to 1989. The map is based on percentiles. The *blank area* in the map refers to the former western part of Berlin

They are likely only to reflect the heteroscedasticity of the underlying SMRs especially for small areas; thus, frequently probability maps are used instead of percentile maps. For the construction of probability maps the O_i are assumed to follow a Poisson distribution with $O_i \sim \text{Po}(\lambda E_i)$ and

$$\Pr(O_i = o_i) = f(o_i, \lambda, E_i) = \frac{e^{-(\lambda E_i)}(\lambda E_i)^{o_i}}{o_i!}. \tag{5.1}$$

Under this assumption the variance of the SMR_i is given by

$$\text{var}(\text{SMR}_i) = \text{var}\left(\frac{o_i}{E_i}\right) = \frac{o_i}{E_i^2} = \frac{\text{SMR}_i}{E_i}. \tag{5.2}$$

In other words the variance is proportional to $\frac{1}{E_i}$. Thus, areas with a small population size tend to give more extreme results. To see this consider an area with $E_i = 0.5$. If we observe one case, the SMR is $1/0.5 = 2$. A further case leads to a SMR of $2/0.5 = 4$. In contrast if $E_i = 5$ and five cases are observed the SMR is $5/5 = 1$. And one additional case will lead to a SMR of $6/5 = 1.25$. This example illustrates that a percentile map of crude SMRs might simply reflect heteroscedasticity between areas and might be misleading.

Probability maps based on Poisson probabilities $\Pr(O_i \geq o_i)$ imply performing a statistical test individually for each region. The parameter λ is given either as the indifference value $\lambda = 1$ or as the maximum likelihood estimate $\hat{\lambda} = \frac{\sum o_i}{\sum E_i}$.

Again, based on this probability map, Fig. 5.3 shows a significant excess in the district of Sebnitz. But probability maps based on a Poisson assumption face the

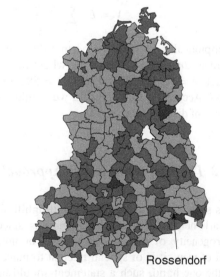

Groups
- ■ SMR>0.99 p<0.05
- ■ SMR>0.99 p>0.05
- ■ SMR<0.99 p>0.05
- □ SMR<0.99 p<0.05

Rossendorf

Fig. 5.3 Childhood leukemia in the former East Germany from 1980 to 1989. The map is based on a significance level with maximum likelihood estimate $\hat{\lambda} = 0.99$

problem of misclassification: Regions with a large population tend to show significant results. Additionally, even if the null hypothesis of constant disease risk is true,
misclassification occurs: Schlattmann and Böhning (1993) showed that probability
maps do not provide a consistent estimate of heterogeneity of disease risk. A false-
positive probability map may cause unnecessary public concern. This is especially
true if a map of a disease such as childhood leukemia is presented, which is attached
to highly emotional effects. Thus, here the question remains of whether the observed
excess risk in the Dresden area is merely a methodological artifact.

In summary, the approaches based on percentile and probability maps are not
particularly helpful. If a Poisson distribution is assumed for the data, overdispersion
frequently occurs. This implies that the variability of the data is much greater than
the variability explained by the model. In other words there is an indication that not
all areas have the same disease risk. A simple of test of overdispersion in disease
maps is the test of Potthoff and Whittinghill (1966). This test is still widely used in
cluster investigations; see, for example, Alexander et al. (1998), Bellec et al. (2006),
or Muirhead (2006). The null hypothesis of this test states

$$H_0: \quad \lambda_1 = \lambda_2 = \cdots = \lambda_n = \lambda, \quad i = 1, n,$$
$$H_A: \quad \lambda_i \sim \Gamma(\alpha, v),$$

where λ_i denotes the area-specific relative risk. The alternative hypothesis states that
area-specific relative risks follow a gamma distribution with scale parameter α and
shape parameter v. Details on the gamma distribution may be found in Sect. 3.2.
Thus, the mean is $\mu = \frac{v}{\alpha}$ and the variance is $\tau^2 = \frac{v}{\alpha^2}$. In other words, under the
alternative hypothesis heterogeneity of disease risks is assumed. The test statistic is
given by

$$V = E_+ \sum_{i=1}^{n} \frac{o_i(o_i - 1)}{E_i}, \quad E_+ = \sum_{i=1}^{n} E_i. \tag{5.3}$$

Asymptotically V follows a normal distribution with expectation $o_+(o_+ - 1)$ and
variance $(2n - 1)o_+ + (o_+ - 1)$, where $o_+ = \sum_{i=1}^{n} o_i$. For the data at hand we obtain $E(V) = 1,332,870$ and $\mathrm{var}(V) = 582,464,190$ with a corresponding z value of
-0.37. According to this result, we would not reject the null hypothesis of homogeneity of disease risk.

5.2.2 The Empirical Bayes Approach

Tests such as that of Potthoff–Whittinghill or tests for autocorrelation are not particularly helpful in cluster investigations, since they only tell the researcher whether
heterogeneity of disease risks exists or not. Furthermore, from a public health
point of view, it is of special interest to make a statement about an individual area.
On the one hand, such a statement should take the variability between areas into
account; on the other hand, it should not lead to spurious elevations of disease risk.

One way to deal with both problems is the use of empirical Bayes methods. The use of empirical Bayes methods for dealing with area-specific relative risks was described by Böhning and Schlattmann (1999), Ugarte et al. (2006), and Ainsworth and Dean (2006).

The Parametric Model

One very flexible approach is given in random effects models, i.e., models where the distribution of relative risks λ_i between areas is assumed to have a probability density function $g(\lambda)$. The O_i are assumed to be Poisson distributed conditional on λ_i with expectation $\lambda_i E_i$.

Several parametric distributions such as the gamma distribution or the log-normal distribution have been suggested for $g(\lambda)$. For details see Clayton and Kaldor (1987) or Mollie and Richardson (1991). A discussion of the choice of the random effects distribution in an empirical Bayes framework was, for example, given by Yasui et al. (2000) and Leyland and Davies (2005).

Among the parametric prior distributions the gamma distribution has been used several times for epidemiologic purposes (Martuzzi and Hills 1995). In the case that the λ_i are assumed to be gamma-distributed, i.e., $\lambda_i \sim \Gamma(\alpha, \nu)$, the parameters α and ν have to be estimated from the data. The marginal distribution is given by

$$\Pr(O_i = o_i) = \int_0^\infty \text{Po}(o_i, \lambda, E_i) g(\lambda) d\lambda, \tag{5.4}$$

where $g(\lambda)$ follows a gamma distribution with scale parameter α and shape parameter ν. Here, we are led to a parametric mixture distribution, namely, the negative binomial distribution (3.6). By applying Bayes's theorem, we can estimate the posterior expectation for the relative risk of the individual area with

$$E(\lambda_i | o_i, \alpha, \nu) = \frac{o_i + \nu}{E_i + \alpha}. \tag{5.5}$$

Proof.

$$\Pr(\lambda_i \leq \lambda | O_i = o_i) = \frac{\Pr(\lambda_i \leq \lambda, O_i = o_i)}{\Pr(O_i = o_i)}$$

$$= \frac{1}{\Pr(O_i = o_i)} \int_0^\lambda f(O_i = o_i, \lambda_i = \theta) f(\theta) d\theta$$

$$= \frac{\int_0^\lambda e^{-\theta E_i} \frac{(\theta E_i)^{o_i}}{o_i!} \frac{\alpha^\nu}{\Gamma(\nu)} \theta^{\nu-1} e^{-\alpha\theta} d\theta}{\binom{\nu+o_i-1}{o_i} \left(\frac{\alpha}{\alpha+E_i}\right)^\nu \left(\frac{E_i}{\alpha+E_i}\right)^{o_i}}$$

$$= \int_0^\lambda e^{-\theta(E_i+\alpha)} \theta^{(o_i+\nu-1)} (E_i + \alpha)^{o_i+\nu} \frac{1}{\Gamma(o_i + \nu)}. \tag{5.6}$$

Thus, the conditional distribution of λ is a gamma distribution with scale parameter $E_i + \alpha$ and shape parameter $o_i + \alpha$. Hence, the mean is given by $\frac{o_i + \nu}{E_i + \alpha}$, which ends the proof. $\square$

Usually α and ν are unknown. Estimates of the parameters α and ν can be obtained either by a method of moments or by combining a method of moments and maximum likelihood estimation. Details of this procedure are given in Sect. 5.5.3.

Note that the empirical Bayes estimates are a compromise between the maximum likelihood estimate of the area-specific relative risk λ with

$$\hat{\lambda}_i = \frac{o_i}{E_i} \tag{5.7}$$

and the mean of the gamma distribution

$$\hat{\mu} = \frac{\hat{\nu}}{\hat{\alpha}}. \tag{5.8}$$

This leads to

$$\hat{\lambda}_i^{\text{EB}} = w_i \frac{o_i}{E_i} + (1 - w_i)\hat{\mu},$$

$$w_i = \left(1 - \frac{\hat{\mu}}{\hat{\tau}^2 E_i}\right)^{-1}, \tag{5.9}$$

where $\hat{\tau}^2 = \frac{\hat{\nu}}{\hat{\alpha}^2}$. As a result, in areas with a large population size the SMR$_i$ based on this empirical Bayes approach changes very little compared with the maximum likelihood estimates, whereas for areas with small population size the SMR$_i$ shrinks to the global mean. On the other hand, if the prior distribution is estimated to have small variance τ^2, this is reflected in a large amount of shrinkage. Thus, parametric empirical Bayes methods provide variance-minimized estimates of the relative risk of the individual area. But these methods still face the problem that they need a post hoc classification of the posterior estimate of the epidemiologic measure to produce maps. Often, this is again done using percentile maps, which may lead to misclassification.

However, as demonstrated in Fig. 5.4 when using the same scale as in Fig. 5.2, we obtain a homogenous map of disease risk of childhood leukemia in the former East Germany. The main distinction between empirical and full Bayesian methods can be seen in the fact that in the case of the empirical Bayes method the parameters of the prior distribution are estimated as point estimates $\hat{\alpha}$ and $\hat{\nu}$ from the data. Thus, the posterior expectation of the relative risk is obtained conditional on these point estimates. In a full Bayesian approach a probability model for the whole set of parameters is specified (including the prior distribution of α and ν) and the posterior expectation of the relative risk is integrated over the posterior distribution of α and ν.

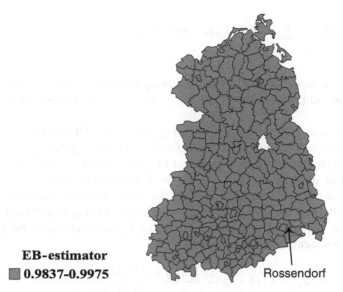

EB-estimator
▨ **0.9837-0.9975**

Rossendorf

Fig. 5.4 Childhood leukemia in the former East Germany from 1980 to 1989. The map is based on a gamma distribution

The Nonparametric Mixture Model Approach

Now let us assume that our population under scrutiny consists of k subpopulations with different levels of disease risk λ_j, $j = 1, \ldots, k$. Each of these subpopulations with disease risk λ_j represents a certain proportion p_j of all regional units. Statistically, this means that the mixing distribution reduces to a finite-mass point distribution. Here we face the problem og identifying the level of risk for each subpopulation and the corresponding proportion of the overall population. One can think of this situation as a *hidden* (or *latent*) structure, since the subpopulation to which each area belongs remains unobserved. These subpopulations may have different interpretations. For example, they could indicate that an important covariate has not been taken into account. Consequently, it is straightforward to introduce an unobserved or latent random vector Z of length k consisting of only 0s besides one 1 at some position (say jth), which then indicates that the area belongs to the jth subpopulation. Taking the marginal density over the unobserved random variable Z, we are led to a discrete semiparametric mixture model. If we assume a nonparametric mixing distribution

$$P = \begin{bmatrix} \lambda_1 & \cdots & \lambda_k \\ p_1 & \cdots & p_k \end{bmatrix} \tag{5.10}$$

for the mixing density $g(\lambda)$ (which can be shown to be always discrete in its nature), we obtain the mixture density as a weighted sum of Poisson densities

$$f(O_i, P, E_j) = \sum_{j=1}^{k} p_j f(O_i, \lambda_j, E_i), \text{ with } \sum_{j=1}^{k} p_j = 1 \text{ and } \geq 0, \ j = 1, \ldots, k.$$

$$(5.11)$$

Note that the model consists of the following parameters: the number of components k, the k unknown relative risks $\lambda_1, \ldots, \lambda_k$, and $k-1$ unknown mixing weights $p_1, \ldots, p_{k-1}$.

For the special case of disease mapping the package DismapWin (Schlattmann 1996) was developed and may be used for this purpose. A general strategy implies calculating the nonparametric maximum likelihood estimator and then applying a backward or forward selection strategy to determine the number of components by means of the likelihood ratio statistic (LRS) (Schlattmann and Böhning 1993). Applying Bayes's theorem and using the estimated mixing distribution as a prior distribution, we are able to compute the probability for each region belonging to a certain component, which is given by

$$\Pr(Z_{ij} = 1 \mid O_i = o_i) = \frac{\Pr(Z_{ij} = 1)\Pr(O_i = o_i \mid Z_{ij} = 1)}{\Pr(O_i = o_i)}. \qquad (5.12)$$

With the parameter estimates obtained from the data this leads to

$$\Pr(Z_{ij} = 1 \mid o_i, \hat{P}, E_i) = \frac{\hat{p}_j f(o_i, \hat{\lambda}_j, E_i)}{\sum\limits_{l=1}^{k} \hat{p}_l f(o_i, \hat{\lambda}_l, E_i)}. \qquad (5.13)$$

The ith area is then assigned to that subpopulation j for which it has the highest posterior probability of belonging. In terms of the latent vector Z Bayes's theorem gives us its posterior distribution. For the leukemia data we find a one-component or homogenous model, with constant disease risk $\hat{\lambda} = 0.99$ and common weight $\hat{p} = 1$. Clearly, in contrast to Figs. 5.2 and 5.3 we obtain a homogenous map for the leukemia data in accordance with Fig. 5.4. The corresponding map is shown in Fig. 5.5. This could also be thought of as using the empirical Bayes estimate based on a posterior distribution which is a constant value for all regions equal to $\hat{\lambda} = \frac{\sum O_i}{\sum E_i}$, in this case.

In general we can compute the posterior expectation for this model as

$$\mathrm{S\hat{M}R}_i = E(\lambda_i \mid o_i, \hat{P}, E_i) = \frac{\sum\limits_{j=1}^{k} \hat{p}_j f(o_i, \hat{\lambda}_j, E_i) \hat{\lambda}_j}{\sum\limits_{l=1}^{k} \hat{p}_l f(o_i, \hat{\lambda}_l, E_i)}. \qquad (5.14)$$

In this special case of a homogenous solution the posterior expectation reduces to the maximum likelihood estimate of the relative risk $\hat{\lambda}$. Results for areas in the vicinity of Rossendorf are listed in Table 5.1. This table contains the crude SMR, the Poisson probability, and empirical Bayes estimates for regions in the Dresden area.

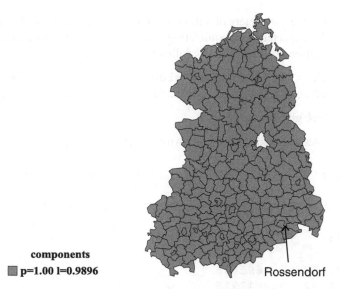

components
■ **p=1.00 l=0.9896**   Rossendorf

Fig. 5.5 Childhood leukemia in the former East Germany from 1980 to 1989. The map is based on a mixture distribution

Table 5.1 Relative risk estimates for areas close to Rossendorf

Area	Cases	Expected cases	SMR	EB	MIX-EB	$\Pr(O \geq o_i)$
Dresden (city)	32	34.41	0.93	0.99	0.99	0.66
Dresden (area)	10	6.8	1.47	0.99	0.99	0.14
Sebnitz	9	3.53	2.55	0.99	0.99	0.01
Pirna	7	7.07	0.99	0.99	0.99	0.55
Bischofswerda	2	4.44	0.45	0.99	0.99	0.93

SMR standardized mortality ratio, *EB* empirical Bayes estimates based on the gamma distribution as a prior distribution, *MIX-EB* posterior expectation of the relative risk based on the mixture distribution

Clearly, looking at Table 5.1 displaying relative risk estimates for areas close to Rossendorf, we conclude that there is no excess risk in the Dresden area on the basis of the spatial resolution of "Landkreise." Further investigations would need to refine the spatial resolution. However, in the case of routine maps produced by a cancer registry we would avoid a false-positive result.

5.3 Computation

Again, we start by loading the package CAMAN and the leukemia data from the former East Germany:

```
> library(CAMAN)
> data(leukDat)
```

In the next step the parameters of a finite mixture model are estimated using a combination of the expectation maximization and vertex exchange method algorithm, that is, the function *mixalg* is used as follows:

```
> mix.leuk <- mixalg(obs="oleuk", pop.at.risk="eleuk",
data=leukDat,family="poisson")
```

Typing *mix.leuk* gives the result

```
Computer Assisted Mixture Analysis:

Data consist of 219 observations (rows).

The Mixture Analysis identified 2 components

DETAILS:
            p        lambda
1  0.00816673  0.1695436
2  0.99183327  0.9943916


Log-Likelihood: -457.3391      BIC: 930.8454
```

Apparently, there is only little heterogeneity present. Thus, we investigate whether a homogenous model is sufficient to describe the data and the expectation maximization algorithm is used to fit a homogenous model.

```
> mix.leuk1<- mixalg.EM(mix.leuk, p=c(1), t= c(1))
```

Typing *mix.leuk1* leads to the shortened output

```
   p    lambda
1  1  0.989624


Log-Likelihood: -457.4043      BIC: 920.1976
```

The corresponding log likelihood is only marginally smaller than that of the initial solution and one would use the homogenous model. However, in order to perform a formal test, a model with components is fit and the parametric bootstrap distribution of the LRS is obtained.

Two calls of the function *mixalg.EM* are possible. The first option implies delivering a *mixalg* object as an argument and providing starting values for the mixing weights and subpopulation means as done in the last call of the function. Alternatively, the data may be given directly together with relevant information such as starting values and the distribution of the mixing kernel. This is shown in the following call of the two-component mixture model:

```
> mix.leuk2<-mixalg.EM(obs="oleuk",pop.at.risk="eleuk",
data=leukDat,family="poisson",p=c(0.01,0.99),
t=c(0.16,0.99))
```

To obtain the distribution of the LRS the function *anova* can be used:

```
> compare<-anova(mix.leuk1,mix.leuk2,nboot=2500)
> compare

  mixture model k      BIC       LL  LL-ratio
1         mix.leuk1 1 920.1976 -457.4043        NA
2         mix.leuk2 2 930.8454 -457.3391 0.1303425

$`LL ratios in bootstrap-data`
     0.9      0.95     0.975       0.99
2.608402 3.862130 5.139111 7.024005
```

Clearly, we do not reject the null hypothesis of a homogenous model. To construct a map, first the map of the former East Germany is loaded:

```
> library(maptools)
> data(GDRmap)
```

Then the map is constructed with the command

```
> plot(GDRmap,col= mix.leuk1@classification)
```

5.4 A Note on Autocorrelation Versus Heterogeneity

Frequently, to assess the "nonrandomness" of a map tests for autocorrelation, e.g., Moran's I (Moran 1948), or heterogeneity, e.g., the test of Potthoff and Whittinghill (1966), are used. The latter accounts for the extra-Poisson variation frequently present in the homogeneous Poisson model. In the following it will be shown that overdispersion can be due to autocorrelation or heterogeneity.

5.4.1 Heterogeneity

Consider a two-level model where the random variable Y has a probability density function $f(y|\lambda)$ with $a \leq y \leq b$. The second level of the model assumes that the parameter λ has probability density function $g(\lambda)$ with $\alpha \leq \lambda \leq \beta$. Under this assumption we are interested in partitioning the unconditional variance $\text{var}(Y)$ into two terms:

$$\text{var}(Y) = E\left[\text{var}(Y|\lambda)\right] + \text{var}\left[E(Y|\lambda)\right]. \tag{5.15}$$

That is, the total variance of Y is decomposed into the variation in the subpopulation with parameter λ and the variation due to the heterogeneity distribution of λ, which is frequently denoted as the heterogeneity variance τ^2. This is sometimes called an analysis of variance with a latent factor. To develop this decomposition we start with the expectation under heterogeneity

$$E(Y) = \int_a^b yf(y)\mathrm{d}y = \int_a^b y \left(\int_\alpha^\beta f(y|\lambda)g(\lambda)\mathrm{d}\lambda \right) \mathrm{d}y$$

$$= \int_\alpha^\beta \left(\int_a^b yf(y|\lambda)\mathrm{d}y \right) g(\lambda)\mathrm{d}\lambda = \int_\alpha^\beta E(Y|\lambda)g(\lambda)\mathrm{d}\lambda$$

$$= E(E(Y|\lambda)). \tag{5.16}$$

The variance $\mathrm{var}(Y)$ is given by

$$\mathrm{var}(Y) = E(Y - E(Y))^2 = \int_a^b (y - E(Y))^2 f(y)\mathrm{d}y$$

$$= \int_a^b (y - E(Y))^2 \left(\int_\alpha^\beta (f(y|\lambda)g(\lambda)\mathrm{d}\lambda \right) \mathrm{d}y$$

$$= \int_a^b (y - \mu(\lambda) + \mu(\lambda) - E(Y))^2 \left(\int_\alpha^\beta f(y|\lambda)g(\lambda)\mathrm{d}\lambda \right) \mathrm{d}y$$

$$= \int_\alpha^\beta \left(\int_a^b (y - \mu(\lambda))^2 f(y|\lambda)\mathrm{d}y \right) g(\lambda)\mathrm{d}\lambda$$

$$+ \int_\alpha^\beta (\mu(\lambda) - E(Y))^2 \left(\int_a^b yf(y|\lambda)\mathrm{d}y \right) g(\lambda)\mathrm{d}\lambda$$

$$= E[\mathrm{var}(Y|\lambda)] + \mathrm{var}[E(Y|\lambda)]. \tag{5.17}$$

This is the well-known result, that the variance of Y is the expectation of the conditional variance of Y plus the variance of the conditional mean of Y; see, e.g., Mood et al. (1974, Chap. V, Theorem 7).

The Poisson Case

For the special case $f(y,\lambda) = \mathrm{Po}(y,\lambda)$ we get $E(Y|\lambda) = \lambda$ and $\mathrm{var}(Y|\lambda) = \lambda$. This leads to the result

$$\mathrm{var}(Y) = E[\mathrm{var}(Y|\lambda)] + \mathrm{var}[E(Y|\lambda)] \tag{5.18}$$

$$= \int_\alpha^\beta \lambda g(\lambda)\mathrm{d}\lambda + \tau^2$$

$$= \mu_\lambda + \tau^2$$

$$= \mu_\lambda + \phi\mu_\lambda$$

$$= \mu_\lambda(1 + \phi). \tag{5.19}$$

5.4.2 Autocorrelation

Suppose that the response variable is the sum of N identically distributed correlated variables X_i, where N itself is a random variable. Given that $Y = X_1 + X_2 + \cdots + X_N$ the expectation $E(Y)$ is given by

$$
\begin{aligned}
E(Y) &= E_N(E_X(X_1 + X_2 \cdots + X_N)) \\
&= E_N(N\mu_X) = \mu_X E(N) = \mu_X \mu_N.
\end{aligned}
\tag{5.20}
$$

This follows from the property of the expectation that $E(\sum X_i) = \sum E(X_i)$. The variance is then given by

$$
\begin{aligned}
\text{var}(Y) &= E_N\left(E_X(Y - \mu_X\mu_N)^2\right) \\
&= E_N\left(E_X(Y - N\mu_X + N\mu_X - \mu_X\mu_N)^2\right) \\
&= E_N\left(E_X(Y - N\mu_X)^2\right) \\
&\quad + 2E_N\left(E_X\left[(Y - N\mu_X)(N\mu_X - \mu_X\mu_N)\right]\right) \\
&\quad + E_N\left(E_X\left[(N\mu_X - \mu_X\mu_N)^2\right]\right).
\end{aligned}
$$

Consider the three terms constituting the variance separately. Starting with

$$
E_N(E_X\left[(Y - N\mu_X)^2\right]) = E_N\left(E_X\left[\left(\sum_{i=1}^N (X_i - \mu_X)\right)^2\right]\right)
$$

and using the standard result

$$
\text{var}\left(\sum_{i=1}^n X_i\right) = \sum_{i=1}^n \text{var}(X_i) + \sum_{i=1}^n \sum_{i \neq j} \text{cov}(X_i, X_j)
$$

leads to

$$
\begin{aligned}
E_N\left(E_X\left[(Y - N\mu_X)^2\right]\right) &= E_N\left(E_X\left[\left(\sum_{i=1}^N (X_i - \mu_X)\right)^2\right]\right) \\
&= E_N\left(N\sigma_X^2 + \sum_{i=1}^n \sum_{i \neq j} \text{cov}(X_i, X_j)\right) \\
&= E_N\left(N\sigma_X^2 + (N^2 - N)\rho\sigma_X^2\right) \\
&= \mu_N\sigma_X^2 + (\sigma_N^2 + \mu_N^2 - \mu_N)\rho\sigma_X^2,
\end{aligned}
\tag{5.21}
$$

where the last line follows from $E(N^2) = \sigma_n^2 + \mu_N^2$.

The next term involves

$$E_N\left(E_X\left[(Y-N\mu_X)(N\mu_X-\mu_N\mu_X)\right]\right)=\mu_X E_N\left[(N-\mu_N)E_X\underbrace{\left(\sum_{i=1}^{N}(X_i-\mu_X)\right)}_{=0}\right]$$

$$=0,$$

since $E_X(X_i-\mu_X)=0$. Finally,

$$E_N\left(E_X\left[(N\mu_X-\mu_X\mu_N)^2\right]\right)=\mu_X^2 E_N\left[(N-\mu_N)^2\right]=\mu_X^2\sigma_N^2. \qquad (5.22)$$

Combining (5.21) and (5.22) gives the variance of the sum of correlated data:

$$\text{var}(Y)=\mu_N\sigma_X^2+(\sigma_N^2+\mu_N^2-\mu_N)\rho\sigma_X^2+\mu_X^2\sigma_N^2. \qquad (5.23)$$

Application to the Poisson Case

First consider the sum of N independent Bernoulli random variables X_i each taking values 0 or 1, where N is assumed to be a Poisson random variable with parameter λ. Then the sum $\sum_{i=1}^{N}X_i$ of Bernoulli variables follows a Poisson distribution with parameter $\lambda\pi$, where $\pi=\Pr(x_i=1)$.

To prove this, consider the probability generating function of an arbitrary discrete random variable Y. If we write $p_k=\Pr(Y=k)$ the probability generating function of Y is given by $G_Y(s)$:

$$G_Y(s)=\sum_{k=0}^{\infty}p_k s^k=E(s^k). \qquad (5.24)$$

For Bernoulli random variables this takes the form

$$G_X(s)=E(s^k)=(1-\pi)s^0+\pi s^1 \qquad (5.25)$$

and for the Poisson distributed random variable the probability generating function is given by

$$\begin{aligned}
G_N(s)&=e^{-\lambda}+s\frac{\lambda e^{-\lambda}}{1!}+s^2\frac{\lambda^2 e^{-\lambda}}{2!}+\cdots\\
&=e^{-\lambda}\left(1+\frac{(s\lambda)^1}{1!}+\frac{(s\lambda)^2}{2!}+\cdots\right)\\
&=e^{-\lambda}e^{s\lambda}\\
&=e^{\lambda(s-1)}.
\end{aligned} \qquad (5.26)$$

Following Feller (1968) the probability generating function of a sum $S_N = X_1 + \cdots + X_N$ of a random number N of independent variables is given by

$$GS_N(s) = G_N(G_X(s)). \tag{5.27}$$

For the problem at hand this leads to

$$
\begin{aligned}
G_N(G_X(s)) &= e^{\lambda(G_X(s)-1)} \\
&= e^{\lambda(1-\pi+\pi s-1)} \\
&= e^{\lambda\pi(s-1)}. \tag{5.28}
\end{aligned}
$$

Thus, $G_N(s)$ is the probability generating function of a Poisson random variable with parameter $\lambda\pi$. Suppose now that we have Poisson count data with $Y = X_1 + X_2 + \cdots + X_N$, with correlated binary random variables, each taking values 0 or 1, then $\Pr(X_i = 1) = \pi$, $\Pr(X_i = 0) = 1 - \pi$, and $\mathrm{Corr}(X_i, X_j) = \rho\,(i \neq j)$.

Coming back to the random sum of correlated Bernoulli data, (5.23) can be used to calculate the variance of these data. The following terms are needed:

$$
\begin{aligned}
\mu_X &= E(X_i) = \pi\,, \\
\sigma_X^2 &= \mathrm{var}(X_i) = \pi(1-\pi)\,, \\
\mu_N &= E(N) = \lambda\,, \\
\sigma_N^2 &= \lambda\,.
\end{aligned}
$$

Thus, $E(Y) = \lambda\pi$ and

$$
\begin{aligned}
\mathrm{var}(Y) &= \lambda\pi(1-\pi) + (\lambda + \lambda^2 - \lambda)\rho\pi(1-\pi) + \pi^2\lambda \\
&= \lambda\pi + \lambda^2\rho\pi(1-\pi) \\
&= \lambda\pi(1+\phi),
\end{aligned}
$$

where $\phi = \lambda\rho(1-\pi)$.

Hence, autocorrelation leads to overdispersion in a similar way as heterogeneity! Thus, heterogeneity models may be used to model correlated count data. However, in the literature there is often the distinction between unstructured and structured heterogeneity. The latter incorporates spatial dependency into the model. One such model is a frequently used Bayesian model which takes a Gaussian random field as an a priori distribution (Besag et al. 1991). In a case study (Schlattmann et al. 1999) it turned out, not surprisingly, that the empirical Bayes methods and full Bayesian methods come to different results. In a large simulation study where the author was involved, it could be shown that the full Bayesian model performed best in most settings (Lawson et al. 2000). However, the second-best performing model was the Poisson–gamma model which is easily used in routine applications, for example, with DismapWin (Schlattmann 1996).

5.5 Focused Clustering

In contrast to general clustering, focused clustering studies investigate the presumably raised incidence of disease in the vicinity of prespecified putative sources of increased risk. As mentioned before, this type of analysis comprises considerable danger of selection bias, since most focused cluster analyses are performed post hoc. There is ongoing public concern with regard to clustering of leukemia in the vicinity of nuclear power plants. Notorious examples are Sellafield in the UK and Krümmel in Germany.

As a result, a large body of statistical methodology was developed to investigate focused clustering. Many of these methods are based on statistical tests where the distance to the point source is considered as a surrogate measure of exposure (Bithell and Stone 1989; Hills and Alexander 1989; Lawson 1993; Stone 1988; Waller et al. 1992). Recently Lawson et al. (2007) proposed a refinement of these methods based on the logistic mode if a control disease is available.

5.5.1 The Score Test for Focused Clustering

The score test by Waller et al. (1992) and Lawson (1993) is widely used in the assessment of focused clustering. Focused cluster tests utilize alternative hypotheses defining increased risk in areas exposed to a focus:

$$
\begin{aligned}
H_0: \quad & E(O_i) = \lambda E_i, \\
H_A: \quad & E(O_i) = \lambda E_i(1 + g_i\beta), \quad i = 1,\ldots,n,
\end{aligned}
\tag{5.29}
$$

where g_i is a function of the distance d_i between the areas considered $(i = 1,\ldots,n)$ and the focus. In the absence of direct exposure data several functions g are used as an exposure surrogate. Note that the additive risk function $1 + g_i\beta$ can be approximated by $\exp\beta$. This follows from the Taylor series expansion (3.19) on page 46 of the function e^β which gives $\exp\beta \approx 1 + \beta g_i$.

The simplest function of exposure is the inverse distance from the source:

$$
g_i = 1/d_i, \quad i = 1,\ldots,n.
\tag{5.30}
$$

Here, distance is computed as the distance from the centroid of the area with coordinates (x_i, y_i) to the focus. Other possible functions are based on exponential functions. See, for example, Tango (2002) for the motivation for the following surrogate measures of exposure:

$$
g_i = \exp(-d_i/\tau), \quad i = 1,\ldots,n, \ \tau > 0 \quad \text{or}
\tag{5.31}
$$
$$
g_i = \exp[-4(d_i/L)^2], \quad i = 1,\ldots,n, \ L > 0.
\tag{5.32}
$$

Figure 5.6 shows a comparison of the three functions. Actually there exist two versions of the score test. These are based on the assumption that the overall relative

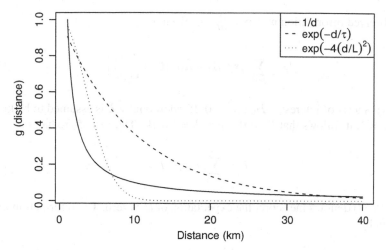

Fig. 5.6 Comparison of three functions of distance as surrogate measures of exposure with $\tau = 10$ and $L = 10$

risk (SMR) is either known or not. For internally standardized data with the whole area as a standard, the overall relative risk λ is unity. In this case the test statistic is given by

$$U^* = \frac{\sum_{i=1}^{n} g_i(o_i - E_i)}{\sqrt{\sum_{i=1}^{n} g_i^2 E_i}}. \tag{5.33}$$

The Score Test as a Special Case of Poisson Regression

The test statistic (5.33) is obtained as a score test based on the likelihood of a Poisson regression model. To see this consider the likelihood of a simple Poisson regression model with logarithmic link function and expected cases E_i as an offset

$$L(\beta) = \prod_{i=1}^{n} \frac{e^{-[\exp(\beta_0 + \beta_1 g_i + \log E_i)]} \exp(\beta_0 + \beta_1 g_i + \log E_i)^{o_i}}{o_i!}.$$

This leads to the following log likelihood function

$$\ell(\beta) = \sum_{i=1}^{n} o_i(\beta_0 + \beta_1 g_i + \log E_i) - \exp(\beta_0 + \beta_1 g_i)E_i - \log(o_i!). \tag{5.34}$$

Taking the derivative of (5.34) with respect to the parameter vector β leads to

$$U(\beta) = \frac{\partial \ell}{\partial \beta} = \sum_{i=1}^{n} [o_i - \exp(\beta_0 + \beta_1 g_i)E_i] \begin{bmatrix} 1 \\ g_i \end{bmatrix}. \tag{5.35}$$

The observed information matrix $-\frac{\partial^2 \ell}{\partial \beta^2}$ is given by

$$I_Y = \sum_{i=1}^{n} [\exp(\beta_0 + \beta_1 g_i) E_i] \begin{bmatrix} 1 & g_i \\ g_i & g_i^2 \end{bmatrix}. \tag{5.36}$$

The hypothesis of interest is $H_0 : \beta_1 = 0$. If, additionally λ is assumed to be known, with $\lambda = 1$, it follows that $\beta_0 = 0$, since $\lambda = \exp \beta_0$. Thus, (5.35) reduces to

$$U = \sum_{i=1}^{n} g_i(o_i - E_i). \tag{5.37}$$

Since (5.37) denotes the score, the expectation of U is zero. The information matrix is given by

$$\frac{\partial^2 \ell}{\partial \beta_1^2} = \sum_{i=1}^{n} g_i^2 E_i. \tag{5.38}$$

Thus, the score test is given by (5.33). If λ is not known, then β_0 is a nuisance parameter which has to estimated. In this case the score test has the form $U_2(\tilde{\beta})^{\mathrm{T}} (I_{f22} - I_{f12} I_{f11}^{-1} I_{f21})^{-1} U_2(\tilde{\beta})$. The mathematical background for this equation is developed in the section "The Score Test for Model Comparison." In particular this is an application of (5.86) developed on page 141. On the basis of this equation the score test is given by

$$T_S = \frac{\left[\sum_{i=1}^{n} g_i(o_i - \hat{\lambda} E_i)\right]^2}{\hat{\lambda} \sum_{i=1}^{n} g_i^2 E_i - (\sum_{i=1}^{n} g_i E_i)^2 / \sum_{i=1}^{n} E_i}, \qquad \hat{\lambda} = \frac{\sum_i o_i}{\sum_i E_i}. \tag{5.39}$$

If $\sum o_i = \sum E_i$, e.g., owing to internal standardization, this reduces to

$$T_S = \frac{\left[\sum_{i=1}^{n} g_i(o_i - E_i)\right]^2}{\sum_{i=1}^{n} g_i^2 E_i - (\sum_{i=1}^{n} g_i E_i)^2 / \sum_{i=1}^{n} E_i}. \tag{5.40}$$

An equivalent form of the test (5.39) is as follows:

$$T_S = \frac{\left[\sum_{i=1}^{n} g_i(o_i - \hat{\lambda} E_i)\right]^2}{\sum_{i=1}^{n} \hat{\lambda} E_i (g_i - \bar{g})^2}, \qquad \bar{g} = \frac{\sum_i g_i E_i}{\sum_i E_i}. \tag{5.41}$$

Note that $\bar{g}$ is a weighted mean of the area's exposure measure. Weights are the expected number of cases in that area. Under H_0, T_S follows a χ^2 distribution with one degree of freedom (Cox and Hinkley 1974, Sect. 9.3).

Example

The apparent excess of cases of childhood leukemia in the village of Seascale near the nuclear reprocessing plant at Sellafield was extensively investigated in the comprehensive report by Black (1984). In addition the focus has also turned to other nuclear installations. For example, Sizewell, a small fishing village in the county of Suffolk, England, located on the East Anglian coast has been under scrutiny. The village itself is overshadowed by two separate nuclear power stations, Sizewell A and Sizewell B. The analysis considers cases of leukemia registered at all ages between 1967 and 1981 in the vicinity of Sizewell within a radius of approximately 17 km. The data were taken from the paper by Bithell and Stone (1989), who applied a Poisson maximum statistic to the data. This test is based on the rank of distances. To use methods based on actual distance, the distance to the power plant was recalculated. In this example inverse distance is used as a surrogate measure of exposure, that is, $g_i = 1/d_i$. According to Fig. 5.7 the relative risk of leukemia apparently decreases with increasing distance from the power plant. Applying the score test (5.41) to the data gives $T_S = 8.332$. Comparing this result with a χ_1^2 distribution leads to a p value of 0.004. Thus, on the basis of this test the null hypothesis is rejected at the 5% level. An association between the distance to the power plant and the relative risk of leukemia might be deduced. However, this result relies on the appropriateness of the Poisson distribution for these data. This is not necessarily the case. Therefore, Sect. 5.5.2 is dedicated to the development and application of more robust versions of the score test.

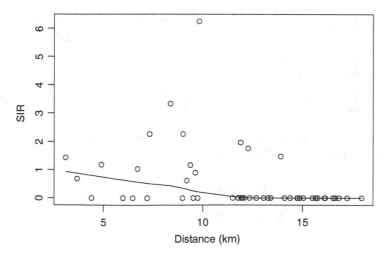

Fig. 5.7 Standardized incidence ratio (*SIR*) of childhood leukemia versus distance to the Sizewell power plant

5.5.2 The Score Test Adjusted for Heterogeneity

The formulation of the score test heavily relies on a Poisson distribution for the data. If the observed cases o_i exhibit overdispersion the variance estimate based on the Fisher information will be too small. Hence, the score test will be anticonservative. Thus, it is desirable to have a form of the score test which allows one to address overdispersion without the need to estimate the parameters of a generalized linear mixed model. A generalized score test is presented consecutively. From (5.96) in the section "Generalized Score Test" the generalized score test is given by

$$T_{GS} = U_2(\hat{\beta})^{\mathrm{T}} V_{GS}^{-1} U_2(\hat{\beta}), \tag{5.42}$$

where $V_{GS} = D_{g22} - I_{g21}I_{g11}^{-1}D_{g21}^{\mathrm{T}} - D_{g21}I_{g11}^{-1}I_{g21}^{\mathrm{T}} + I_{g21}I_{g11}^{-1}D_{g11}I_{g11}^{-1}I_{g21}^{\mathrm{T}}$. The observed information is contained in (5.36). The matrix D_Y is given by

$$D_Y = \sum_{i=1}^{n} [o_i - \exp(\beta_0 + \beta_1 g_i)E_i]^2 \begin{bmatrix} 1 & g_i \\ g_i & g_i^2 \end{bmatrix}. \tag{5.43}$$

Thus, the variance V_{GS} evaluated at $\beta_1 = 0$ with $\hat{\lambda} = \exp(\hat{\beta}_0) = \frac{\sum o_i}{\sum E_i}$ is given by

$$
\begin{aligned}
V_{GS} &= \sum (o_i - \hat{\lambda} E_i)^2 g_i^2 - \frac{\hat{\lambda} \sum E_i g_i \sum (o_i - \hat{\lambda})^2 g_i}{\hat{\lambda} \sum E_i} \\
&\quad - \frac{\sum (o_i - \hat{\lambda})^2 g_i \hat{\lambda} \sum E_i g_i}{\hat{\lambda} \sum E_i} + \frac{\hat{\lambda}^2 \sum_{i=1} (o_i - \hat{\lambda} E_i)^2 (\sum E_i g_i)^2}{\hat{\lambda}^2 (\sum E_i)^2} \\
&= \sum (o_i - \hat{\lambda} E_i)^2 g_i^2 - 2 \times \frac{\sum (o_i - \hat{\lambda})^2 g_i \sum E_i g_i}{\sum E_i} + \frac{\sum (o_i - \hat{\lambda} E_i)^2 (\sum E_i g_i)^2}{(\sum E_i)^2} \\
&= \sum \left(g_i - \frac{\sum g_i E_i}{\sum E_i} \right)^2 (o_i - \hat{\lambda} E_i)^2 \\
&= \sum (g_i - \bar{g})^2 (o_i - \hat{\lambda} E_i)^2, \quad \bar{g} = \frac{\sum_i g_i E_i}{\sum_i E_i}.
\end{aligned} \tag{5.44}
$$

In contrast to (5.41), the model-based variance is replaced by the empirical variance (without the denominator). This leads to the test statistic

$$T_{GS} = \frac{\left[\sum_{i=1}^{n} g_i (o_i - \hat{\lambda} E_i) \right]^2}{\sum_{i=1}^{n} (g_i - \bar{g})^2 (o_i - \hat{\lambda} E_i)^2}, \quad \bar{g} = \frac{\sum_i g_i E_i}{\sum_i E_i}. \tag{5.45}$$

Example Revisited

Coming back to the example and applying the generalized score test given by (5.45) leads to a value of the test statistic $T_{GS} = 2.9755$. Comparing this result with a χ_1^2

distribution leads to a p value of 0.0846. Thus, if we allow for misspecification of the model, the null hypothesis is no longer rejected at the 5% level. This is in accordance with the result of Bithell and Stone (1989). Using Stone's test, they also found that

> The Sizewell data are altogether less statistically significant. Geographical proximity to the nuclear power station does not seem to be particularly important.

5.5.3 The Score Test Based on the Negative Binomial Distribution

Here, the parameterization as in (3.25) is used. This leads to the likelihood

$$L(\beta, v) = \prod_{i=1}^{n} \frac{\Gamma(o_i + v)}{\Gamma(o_i)\Gamma(v)} \left[\frac{v}{\exp(\beta_0 + \beta_1 g_i)E_i + v} \right]^v \left[\frac{\exp(\beta_0 + \beta_1 g_i)E_i}{\exp(\beta_0 + \beta_1 g_i)E_i + v} \right]^{o_i}.$$

(5.46)

Since

$$\frac{\Gamma(y+c)}{\Gamma(c)} = c(c+1) + \cdots + (c+y-1), \quad c > 0, \ y \in \mathbb{N},$$

(5.47)

as shown by Lawless (1987), the log likelihood function is given by

$$\ell(\beta, v) = \sum_{i=1}^{n} \left(\sum_{j=0}^{o_i-1} \log(1 + vj) + v \log(v) - (o_i + v) \log(\lambda_i E_i + v) + o_i \log(\lambda_i E_i) \right),$$

(5.48)

where $\lambda_i = \exp(\beta_0 + \beta_1 g_i)$. Taking the derivative with respect to the parameter vector β leads to

$$U(\beta) = \frac{\partial \ell}{\partial \beta} = v \sum_{i=1}^{n} \left[\frac{o_i - \lambda_i E_i}{v + \lambda_i E_i} \right] \begin{bmatrix} 1 \\ g_i \end{bmatrix}.$$

(5.49)

Hence, the observed information matrix is given by

$$I_Y = v \sum_{i=1}^{n} \left[\lambda_i E_i \frac{o_i + v}{(\lambda_i E_i + v)^2} \right] \begin{bmatrix} 1 & g_i \\ g_i & g_i^2 \end{bmatrix}.$$

(5.50)

Again, the variance estimate based on the observed information matrix is given by

$$\text{var}(U) = I_{Y22} - I_{Y12} I_{Y11}^{-1} I_{Y21}.$$

(5.51)

Thus, the variance of the score evaluated at $\beta_1 = 0$ is obtained as

$$\text{var}(U) = v\lambda \left[\sum_{i=1}^{n} \frac{g_i^2 E_i (o_i + v)}{(\lambda E_i + v)^2} - \frac{\left(\sum_{i=1}^{n} \frac{g_i E_i (o_i + v)}{(\lambda E_i + v)^2} \right)^2}{\sum_{i=1}^{n} \frac{(o_i + v) E_i}{(\lambda E_i + v)^2}} \right].$$

(5.52)

Considering I_{Y11} and replacing $\lambda = \frac{v}{\alpha}$ leads to

$$\sum_{i=1}^{n} \frac{(o_i + v)E_i}{(\lambda E_i + v)^2} = \sum_{i=1}^{n} \frac{(o_i + v)E_i}{(\frac{v}{\alpha})^2(E_i + \alpha)^2}$$

$$= \frac{1}{\lambda^2} \sum_{i=1}^{n} \frac{\hat{\theta}_i E_i}{E_i + \alpha}, \quad \text{since } \hat{\theta}_i = \frac{o_i + v}{E_i + \alpha}. \tag{5.53}$$

Thus, expressing the observed information in terms of the empirical Bayes estimators $\hat{\theta}_i$ simplifies the presentation considerably. Additionally, defining $E_i^* = 1/(1 + \frac{\alpha}{E_i})$ allows us to write (5.52) as

$$\text{var}(U) = \alpha \left[\sum_{i=1}^{n} g_i^2 \hat{\theta}_i E_i^* - \frac{(\sum_{i=1}^{n} g_i \hat{\theta}_i E_i^*)^2}{\sum_{i=1}^{n} \hat{\theta}_i E_i^*} \right]$$

$$= \alpha \sum_{i=1}^{n} \hat{\theta} E_i^* (g_i - \bar{g})^2, \quad \bar{g} = \frac{\sum g_i \hat{\theta}_i E_i^*}{\sum \hat{\theta}_i E_i^*}. \tag{5.54}$$

Since α and v are not known they need to be estimated from the data as outlined in Sect. 5.5.4. Using (5.54), we obtain the score test statistic based on the negative binomial distribution as

$$T_{\text{SNB}} = \frac{\hat{v}^2}{\hat{\alpha}} \frac{\left[\sum_{i=1}^{n} \frac{g_i(o_i - \hat{\lambda} E_i)}{v + \lambda E_i} \right]^2}{\sum_{i=1}^{n} \hat{\theta}_i E_i^* (g_i - \bar{g})^2}, \quad \bar{g} = \frac{\sum g_i \hat{\theta}_i E_i^*}{\sum \hat{\theta} E_i^*}. \tag{5.55}$$

This test statistic is quite similar to (5.41). The weighted mean $\bar{g}$ is again a weighted mean of the individual area's surrogate exposure measure, weighted with the pseudo expected number of cases E_i^* and the empirical Bayes estimates $\hat{\theta}_i$ in that area. Under H_0, T_{SNB} follows again asymptotically a χ^2 distribution with one degree of freedom (Cox and Hinkley 1974).

5.5.4 Estimation of α and v

Finally, the unknown parameters α and v need to be replaced with their estimates. Here the method proposed by Clayton and Kaldor (1987) and a method of moments is applied. The method by Clayton and Kaldor combines maximum likelihood and method of moments estimation. We start with the log likelihood. For the case of no covariates the log likelihood function (5.48) reduces to

$$\ell(\beta, v) = \sum_{i=1}^{n} \left[\sum_{j=0}^{o_i - 1} \log(1 + vj) + v \log \alpha - (o_i + v) \log(E_i + \alpha) \right]. \tag{5.56}$$

Equating the first derivative of (5.56) with respect to α to zero leads to the equation

$$\frac{\hat{v}}{\hat{\alpha}} = \frac{1}{n}\sum_{i=1}^{n}\frac{o_i+\hat{v}}{E_i+\hat{\alpha}} = \frac{1}{n}\sum_{i=1}^{n}\hat{\theta}_i. \qquad (5.57)$$

Next, equating the sum of the squared Pearson residuals r_P to its asymptotic expectation $(n-1)$ leads to a moment estimate for the variance of the mixing distribution. Here r_P is given by

$$r_P = \frac{o_i - \hat{\lambda}E_i}{\sqrt{\frac{\hat{v}}{\hat{\alpha}}E_i + E_i^2\frac{\hat{v}}{\hat{\alpha}^2}}}. \qquad (5.58)$$

Solving for the heterogeneity variance $\frac{v}{\alpha^2}$ leads to

$$\frac{\hat{v}}{\hat{\alpha}^2} = \frac{1}{n-1}\sum_{i=1}^{n}\left(1+\frac{\hat{\alpha}}{E_i}\right)(\hat{\theta}_i-\hat{\lambda})^2. \qquad (5.59)$$

Set starting values for $\hat{\alpha}^{(0)} = 1$ and $\hat{v}^{(0)} = 1$
Step 1: Compute $\kappa_1 = \frac{\hat{v}}{\hat{\alpha}} = \sum_{i=1}^{n}\hat{\theta}_i$
Step 2: Find $\kappa_2 = \frac{v}{\hat{\alpha}^2} = \frac{1}{n-1}\sum_{i=1}^{n}\left(1+\frac{\hat{\alpha}}{E_i}\right)(\hat{\theta}_i-\frac{\hat{v}}{\hat{\alpha}})^2$
Step 3: Set $\hat{\alpha}^{(l)} = \frac{\kappa_1}{\kappa_2}$ and $\hat{v}^{(l)} = \frac{\kappa_1^2}{\kappa_2}$ and go to step 1

Algorithm 5.5.1: Combined moment and maximum likelihood estimator algorithm for the estimation of the parameters of the negative binomial distribution

Thus, Algorithm 5.5.1 for the computation of $\hat{\alpha}$ and $\hat{v}$ is obtained. The algorithm is usually stopped when two consecutive estimates are close to each other, where closeness is defined by some value ε. Here ε is taken to be 0.00001. Usually this algorithm converges very fast, i.e., after five iterations. However, if the amount of heterogeneity between areas is small, the algorithm sometimes fails to converge and the iteration jumps back and forth between two points. To avoid this complication a moment estimator is considered for the dispersion parameter v. In simulation studies for simple count data conducted by Saha and Paul (2005) the moment estimator based on the sample mean $\bar{x}$ and the sample variance S^2

$$\hat{v} = \frac{\bar{x}^2}{S^2 - \bar{x}} \qquad (5.60)$$

has acceptable properties in terms of bias and variance. Applying the general result $\text{var}(Y) = E[\text{var}(Y|\lambda)] + \text{var}[E(Y|\lambda)]$ to the negative binomial distribution and taking the number of expected cases E into account leads to

$$\text{var}(O) = \lambda E + \frac{\lambda^2}{v}E^2. \qquad (5.61)$$

Now we consider a random sample $O_1, \ldots, O_n$ with $i = 1, \ldots, n$ and corresponding expected cases $E_1, E_2, \ldots, E_n$. Assuming independence yields an estimate of the
variance

$$\sum \text{var}(O_i) = \lambda \sum E_i + \frac{\lambda^2}{\nu} \sum E_i^2. \tag{5.62}$$

Replacing $\text{var}(O_i)$ by $(O_i - \lambda E_i)^2$ and solving for ν leads to the following estimator
for ν

$$\hat{\nu} = \frac{\lambda^2 \sum E_i^2}{\sum (o_i - \lambda E_i)^2 - \lambda \sum E_i}. \tag{5.63}$$

Usually λ is not known and needs to be estimated from the data too. Here the arith-
metic mean of the SMR_i is used:

$$\hat{\lambda} = \frac{1}{N} \sum \frac{o_i}{E_i}. \tag{5.64}$$

Now, an estimate for α is obtained by

$$\hat{\alpha} = \frac{\hat{\nu}}{\hat{\lambda}} \tag{5.65}$$

Example Revisited

Coming back to the example of childhood leukemia in the vicinity of the Sizewell
power plant, we obtain an estimate $\hat{\nu} = 0.369$. With $\hat{\lambda} = 0.547$ the estimate of $\hat{\alpha}$ is
given by 0.675. Finally, applying the test statistic (5.55) leads to $T_{\text{SNB}} = 2.247$ with
a corresponding p value of 0.1334. Again, on the basis of this result, geographic
proximity to Sizewell does not seem to be an important risk factor for leukemia.
Both score tests which allow for heterogeneity between areas do not suggest that
proximity to Sizewell is of major concern. The initial association based on the standard Poisson score test might be the result of unobserved confounding factors, such
as social deprivation. Taking unobserved heterogeneity into account results in different conclusions.

5.6 Case Study: Leukemia in Adults in the Vicinity of Krümmel

Hoffmann and Schlattmann (1999)[2] analyzed the association between leukemia
in adults and proximity to the nuclear power plant at Krümmel in the northern
part of Germany. Figure 5.8 shows the location of the power plant. The above-
mentioned authors found no association between leukemia and proximity to the
power plant. This case study provides a partial reanalysis of these data of Hoffmann
and Schlattmann (1999) applying the newly developed score tests and covariate-
adjusted mixture models.

---

[2] The use of part of the material in this book is kindly permitted by John Wiley & Sons.

Fig. 5.8 Geographic location of the "Kernkraftwerk Krümmel" in northern Germany (the diameter of the *circle* represents approximately 30 km)

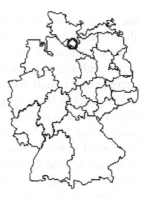

5.6.1 Background

Between February 1990 and the end of the year 1995 six cases of childhood leukemia were diagnosed among residents of the small rural community of Elbmarsch in northern Germany. Five of these cases were diagnosed in only 16 months between February 1990 and May 1991 (Dieckmann 1992). All patients lived in close proximity (500–4,500 m) to Germany's largest capacity nuclear boiling water reactor, the 1,300-MW (electric) Kernkraftwerk Krümmel. This plant was commissioned in 1984. It is situated on the northern bank of the Elbe, a major river which separates Schleswig-Holstein and Lower Saxony. Standardized incidence ratios for childhood leukemia in a circular area with a radius of 5 km around the plant were 4.60 (95% confidence interval 2.10–10.30) for the time period 1990–1995 and 11.80 (95% confidence interval 4.90–28.30) if the analysis is restricted to the years 1990 and 1991, respectively (Hoffmann et al. 1997). From January 1, 1996 until 1998, three additional childhood leukemia cases have been confirmed in the 5-km area around the plant, rendering the magnitude of the childhood leukemia cluster in Elbmarsch unprecedented worldwide with respect to the number of cases together with the narrow spatial and brief temporal dimension. It initiated a large body of ongoing research based on data of the German childhood cancer registry; see, for example, Michaelis et al. (1992), Michaelis (1998), or Kaatsch et al. (1998, 2008).

Soon after the cluster had been identified, the governments of Lower Saxony and Schleswig-Holstein established boards of experts to advise on useful investigations and appropriate methods to identify possible causes for the cluster. The board's members' scientific backgrounds included hematology, pediatrics, toxicology, radiobiology, medical physics, geology, virology, statistics, public health, and epidemiology. An extended array of established or suspected risk factors have been investigated. However, measurements of outdoor and indoor air, soil, drinking water, private wells, milk, vegetables, other garden products, and mushrooms for heavy metals, organochlorine compounds, benzene, toluene, and aromatic amines, respectively, did not reveal any clue indicative of unusual contamination. An indoor-air radon concentration of 610 Bq m^{-3} was measured inside the home of one child, but not in the homes of the other children. Moreover, this activity was only slightly above the current recommendation for existing houses in Germany. A thorough review of medical and hospital records, and extensive semistructured personal interviews with the afflicted families failed to reveal any unusual dose of medical or occupational radiation or exposure to cytostatic or other leukemogenic drugs. None of the children had a preexisting medical condition known to be associated with a higher risk of leukemia. All children were born in the local area and most of the parents had lived there for many years prior to the children's births. Despite this residential stability, none of the patients' families were found to be related to any of the others and the afflicted children had not had direct contact with each other prior to their diagnoses. Biological samples (breast milk, urine, blood) taken from members of the afflicted families and other inhabitants of Elbmarsch yielded low background values of 2,3,7,8-TCDD, various organochlorines, lead, and cadmium. The prevalence of antibodies against viruses that are discussed as potentially leukemogenic was below the German average, if any were present. At this point both boards of experts came to the conclusion that further investigations on the basis of only the diseased children and their families would hardly shed much more light on the cause of the cluster. Instead, a comprehensive retrospective incidence study was suggested which should cover all ages, a sufficiently large study area, and a sufficient time period to generate a study base suited for an analytic epidemiologic investigation.

5.6.2 The Retrospective Incidence Study Elbmarsch

A retrospective incidence study ("Retrospective Incidence Study Elbmarsch"; RIS-E) was conducted between November 1992 and August 1994. The study region included three counties adjacent to the nuclear power plant, i.e., the counties of Lüneburg and Harburg in Lower Saxony and the county of Herzogtum Lauenburg in Schleswig-Holstein. The total study population was about 470,000. Case ascertainment included all leukemias, malignant lymphomas, and multiple myelomas as well as the myelodysplastic and myeloproliferative syndromes (ICD-9 200-208, 238.7), covering the 10-year period from 1984 to 1993.

Leukemia cases were categorized as acute and chronic leukemia, respectively, according to the Ninth International Classification of Diseases (German version). This case study is restricted to chronic leukemia in men since this was the only category with a hint of an association between the disease and the power plant.

Inclusion criteria were (1) first diagnosis of a target disease in the study period, (2) place of residence within the study area at the time of first diagnosis, and (3) German citizenship. Since no epidemiologic cancer registry exists in Lower Saxony and Schleswig-Holstein, cases had to be ascertained exclusively from primary data sources. Extraction was based exclusively on original documents.

For calculation of incidence rates, population figures for all of the 217 rural communities of the study area were provided by the State Statistical Offices of Lower

Saxony and of Schleswig-Holstein by 5-year age groups, gender, and citizenship for the whole observation period from 1984 to 1992. One of the rural communities was uninhabited over the entire study period. All analyses presented in this section are based on 216 geographical units representing rural communities which contributed to the denominator. Population data for 1992 were substituted for population data for 1993.

For the purposes of the analyses presented here, rural communities were used as the unit of observation; hence all incident cases were assigned to the community of residence of the patients at the time of their first diagnosis. The number of expected cases were then calculated using the total number of incident cases in the study area and each community's respective fraction of age-specific population years at risk.

In this case study we simply deal with the point source of the nuclear power plant at Krümmel; hence, we predominantly investigate a focused clustering problem. Nevertheless, we feel that an analysis of general clustering is also necessary since the use of disease maps based on (empirical) Bayes models allows us to separate signal from noise in the geographic distribution of disease within small areas. A thorough description of the data is given in the article by Hoffmann and Schlattmann (1999).

5.6.3 Focused Analysis

For the focused analysis we start with the traditional descriptive approach of calculating the standardized incidence ratio for each concentric region together with a 95% confidence interval, the latter being calculated using Byar's method as described by Breslow and Day (1987, Chap. 2, p. 69). On the basis of the results shown in Table 5.2, there seems to be an excess risk of chronic leukemia for men within the first circle closest to the power plant. This might be a spurious association. Another choice of circles might lead to different results! Implicitly many statistical tests are performed, which leads to the problem of multiple comparisons. Thus, tests using all the information should be preferred. According to the results from the disease mapping in Sect. 5.6.4 there is overdispersion present. That is why the extensions of the standard score test developed in the previous sections are called for.

Table 5.2 Chronic leukemia in men: traditional method

Distance (km)	o_i	E_i	SIR	95% CI
<5	20	11.74	1.70	1.03–2.63
5 < 10	9	10.23	0.88	0.40–1.67
10 < 15	26	32.35	0.80	0.52–1.18
15 < 20	24	33.25	0.72	0.46–1.07
≥20	118	109.41	1.07	0.89–1.29

SIR standardized incidence ratio, *CI* confidence interval

Table 5.3 Results of the score and generalized score tests for chronic leukemia in men in the vicinity of Krümmel

Test	T_S	T_{GS}	T_{NBS}
Value	1.96	0.451	0.339
p	0.162	0.520	0.560

In assessing the association between the distance to the power plant we restrict our analysis to the function of distance $g(d) = \exp(-d_i/L)^2$, with $L = 10$. The reason for doing so is that in the analysis by Hoffmann and Schlattmann (1999) only this function suggested a potential association between the power plant and chronic leukemia in men. The results displayed in Table 5.3 do not indicate that geographic proximity to the power plant should be of concern. Using other functions of distance, such as inverse distance, does not change the results.

5.6.4 Disease Mapping and Model-Based Methods

In their case study Hoffmann and Schlattmann (1999) found a homogeneous distribution of disease risk for acute leukemias in men and women, whereas for chronic leukemias heterogeneity of disease risk was present. For chronic leukemias we obtain a two-component solution for both men and women. For men, the two-component solution has a log likelihood of -165.895 compared with a log likelihood of -168.18 for the homogenous solution. The LRS is 4.56, with a 95% simulated critical value of 4.01; therefore, we accept the two-component model.

Looking at the map in Fig. 5.9 it becomes clear that there are "low-risk" and "high risk" areas; however "high-risk" areas do not seem to be concentrated in the vicinity of the power plant. To investigate this impression more formally, a natural extension of the model is to include a distance-based covariate. In the simplest case of the homogenous model a Poisson regression model with *offset* $\log E_i$ is considered. This implies that $\log E_i$ in the linear predictor

$$\eta_i = \beta_0 + \beta_1 g(d_i) + \log E_i \tag{5.66}$$

has a fixed regression coefficient equal to unity. Again, this model can be extended to covariate-adjusted finite mixture models (Schlattmann et al. 1996). The expectation of the ith observation in the jth subpopulation is then given by

$$E(O_{ij}) = \exp(\beta_{0j} + \beta_{1j}x_{i1} + \cdots + \beta_{mj}x_{im})E_i. \tag{5.67}$$

This leads to the mixture density

$$f(o_i, \lambda_j, E_i) = \sum_{j=1}^{k} p_j f(o_i, \lambda_j, E_i). \tag{5.68}$$

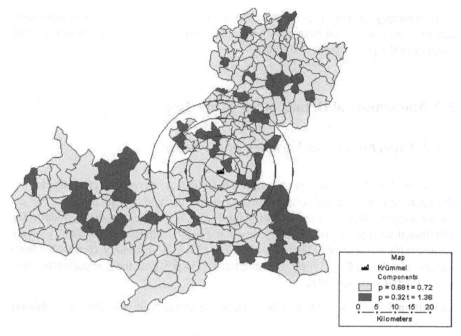

Fig. 5.9 Map of chronic leukemia in men: incidence in the vicinity of Krümmel

Table 5.4 Poisson and covariate-adjusted mixture model for chronic leukemia in men with a function $g(d)$ of distance to the power plant as a covariate

k	Parameter	Weight p_j	Estimate	Standard error	$\log L$
1	Intercept	1	0.000		-168.180
1	Intercept	1	-0.025	0.074	-167.430
	$g(d) = \exp(-d_i/10)^2$	–	0.673	0.484	
2	Intercept 1	0.6	-0.329	0.119	-165.895
	Intercept 2	0.4	0.305	0.085	
2	Intercept 1	0.575	-0.345	0.121	-165.559
	Intercept 2	0.425	0.266	0.021	
	$g(d) = \exp(-d_i/10)^2$	–	0.404	0.519	

Using this class of models and looking for a parsimonious model, we find on the basis of the results in Table 5.4 that there is no association between the occurrence of leukemia and the distance to the power plant. Comparing the homogenous models with and without the distance-based covariate, the LRS is 1.5 and thus the null hypothesis is not rejected. When heterogeneity is taken into account by using a covariate-adjusted finite mixture model, the value of the likelihood ratio test for the effect of distance is 0.672. Comparing this with a χ_1^2 distribution does not lead to the rejection of the null hypothesis!

In summary, on the basis these data using a variety of methods there is no indication of an association between chronic leukemia in men and living in the close vicinity of the power plant at Krümmel.

5.7 Mathematical Details of the Score Test

5.7.1 Expectation and Variance of the Score

The score U is of fundamental importance in statistical inference. Before developing the score test, we determine the expectation and the variance of the score. To do so we suppose that the random variables $Y_1, \ldots, Y_n$ are independently identically distributed with probability density function $f(y_i|\theta)$, where θ is potentially vector valued with m elements. Then $Y = (Y_1, Y_2, \ldots, Y_n)$ is absolutely continuous with density $p(y|\theta) = \prod_{i=1}^n f(y_i|\theta)$. For simplicity of exposition, the one-parameter case is considered subsequently.

Definition 5.2. The score U of Y is given by the first derivative of the log likelihood function:

$$U(Y|\theta) = \frac{\partial \log p(Y|\theta)}{\partial \theta}. \qquad (5.69)$$

Proposition 5.1. *The score $U(Y|\theta)$ has expectation $E(U(Y|\theta)) = 0$.*

Proof. Since $p(y|\theta)$ is a probability density function $\int p(y|\theta)dy = 1$. Assuming exchangeability of differentiation and integration leads to

$$\int p(y|\theta)dy = 1 \Leftrightarrow \frac{\partial}{\partial \theta} \int p(y|\theta)dy = 0 \Leftrightarrow \int \frac{\partial p(y|\theta)}{\partial \theta} \frac{1}{p(y|\theta)} p(y|\theta)dy$$

$$= \int \frac{\partial \log p(y|\theta)}{\partial \theta} p(y|\theta)dy$$

$$= E(U(Y|\theta)) = 0. \qquad (5.70)$$

$\square$

As a result, the variance of the score is given by

$$\mathrm{var}\,(U(Y|\theta)) = E(U(Y|\theta)^2) - E(U(Y|\theta))^2 = E(U(Y|\theta)^2). \qquad (5.71)$$

Proposition 5.2. *The variance of the score* $\mathrm{var}\,(U)$ *is given by the expected Fisher information* $I_{\mathrm{f}}(\theta) = -E\left(\frac{\partial^2 \log p(y|\theta)}{\partial \theta^2}\right)$.

Proof. Differentiating (5.70) leads to

$$0 = \frac{\partial}{\partial\theta}\left(\int \frac{\partial \log p(y|\theta)}{\partial\theta} p(y|\theta)dy\right) \Leftrightarrow \tag{5.72}$$

$$0 = \int \frac{\partial \log p(y|\theta)}{\partial\theta}\frac{\partial p(y|\theta)}{\partial\theta}dy + \int \frac{\partial^2 \log p(y|\theta)}{\partial\theta^2} p(y|\theta)dy \Leftrightarrow \tag{5.73}$$

$$\int \left(\frac{\partial \log p(y|\theta)}{\partial\theta}\right)^2 p(y|\theta)dy = -\int \frac{\partial^2 \log p(y|\theta)}{\partial\theta^2} p(y|\theta)dy \Leftrightarrow \tag{5.74}$$

$$E(U^2) = -E\left(\frac{\partial^2 \log p(y|\theta)}{\partial\theta^2}\right) = I_f(\theta) \Leftrightarrow \tag{5.75}$$

$$\text{var}(U) = I_f(\theta) \text{ with } (5.71). \tag{5.76}$$

□

5.7.2 The Score Test

The Score Test as a Likelihood Ratio Test

Theoretical development of the score test may be found in Cox and Hinkley (1974, Sect. 9.3). It is reviewed in part in this section as far as necessary for the development of generalized score tests. For simplicity the one-parameter notation is used. In the following, the score test is developed as an approximation to the likelihood ratio test given by

$$e^{\frac{1}{2}W} = \frac{L(\hat{\theta}\,|\,Y)}{L(\theta_0\,|\,Y)}. \tag{5.77}$$

On the log scale this results in

$$W = 2(\log L(\hat{\theta}\,|\,Y) - \log L(\theta_0\,|\,Y). \tag{5.78}$$

Now the first term is expanded as

$$\log L(\hat{\theta}\,|\,Y) = \log L(\theta_0\,|\,Y) + (\hat{\theta} - \theta_0)U(\hat{\theta}) + \frac{1}{2}(\hat{\theta} - \theta_0)^2\frac{\partial U}{\partial\theta_0} + o_p(1), \tag{5.79}$$

where $o_p(1)$ denotes a quantity that converges to 0 in probability. Then,

$$W = 2(\log L(\theta_0\,|\,Y) - \log L(\theta_0\,|\,Y) - (\hat{\theta} - \theta_0)U(\hat{\theta}) - \frac{1}{2}(\hat{\theta} - \theta_0)^2\frac{\partial U}{\partial\theta_0} + o_p(1)$$

$$= -(\hat{\theta} - \theta_0)^2\frac{\partial U}{\partial\theta_0} + o_p(1)$$

$$= (\hat{\theta} - \theta_0)^2 I_f(\theta_0) + o_p(1).$$

The score $U(\hat{\theta})$ can be expanded by a Taylor series as follows:

$$U(\hat{\theta}) = U(\theta_0) + \frac{\partial U(\theta)}{\partial \theta}(\hat{\theta} - \theta_0) + o_p(1). \tag{5.80}$$

Thus, since $U(\hat{\theta}) = 0$ it follows that

$$(\hat{\theta} - \theta_0) = I_f^{-1}(\theta_0)U(\theta_0) + o_p(1). \tag{5.81}$$

Substituting (5.81) into (5.80) gives the score statistic (Rao 1948) for the multi-parameter case as

$$W = U(\theta_0)^{\mathrm{T}} I_f^{-1}(\theta_0)U(\theta_0) + o_p(1). \tag{5.82}$$

The Score Test for Model Comparison

Suppose we have a set of observations whose log likelihood function depends on an unknown parameter vector $\theta = (\theta_1, \ldots, \theta_m)^{\mathrm{T}}$. Then the score test can then be used for model comparison (McCullagh and Nelder 1989). Consider two models, one (M_1) with r_1 and a second extended model (M_2) with $m = r_1 + r_2$ parameters. Comparison of these two models can be performed with the LRS, the Wald test, and the score test. All these tests are asymptotically equivalent. In contrast to the Wald test, the LRS and the score test are invariant to transformations, which makes these tests more attractive. Comparing the LRS and the score test, we find that the latter is computationally less expensive and is therefore of special interest in some applications.

To consider the properties of the score test in more detail let $\ell(y, \theta_1, \theta_2)$ be a log likelihood function depending on a response vector y and parameter vector $\theta :=$ (θ_1, θ_2). We wish to test the composite hypothesis $H_0 : \theta_2 = 0$ versus the alternative that θ_2 is unrestricted. Here, θ_2 corresponds to the additional parameters in model M_2. The components of θ_1 are called nuisance parameters since they are not of interest in the test for θ_2. But, nevertheless the parameters θ_1 need to be estimated in order to perform the test.

The partitioned vector $\theta^{\mathrm{T}} = (\theta_1^{\mathrm{T}}, \theta_2^{\mathrm{T}})$ leads to a simple form of Rao's test, where the partitioned vector is given by

$$U = \frac{\partial \ell}{\partial \theta} = \left(\underbrace{\frac{\partial \ell}{\partial \theta_{11}}, \ldots, \frac{\partial \ell}{\partial \theta_{1r_1}}}_{U_1}, \underbrace{\frac{\partial \ell}{\partial \theta_{21}}, \ldots, \frac{\partial \ell}{\partial \theta_{2m}}}_{U_2} \right). \tag{5.83}$$

If $\hat{\theta}$ is the maximum likelihood estimate of the restricted model, then

$$U_1(\hat{\theta}) = 0. \tag{5.84}$$

The Fisher information I_f is given by

$$I_f = \begin{bmatrix} -E\left(\frac{\partial U_1^T}{\partial \theta_1}\right) & -E\left(\frac{\partial U_1^T}{\partial \theta_2}\right) \\ -E\left(\frac{\partial U_2^T}{\partial \theta_1}\right) & -E\left(\frac{\partial U_2^T}{\partial \theta_2}\right) \end{bmatrix} = \begin{bmatrix} I_{f11} & I_{f12} \\ I_{f21} & I_{f22} \end{bmatrix}. \tag{5.85}$$

Then (5.82) with $U_2(\theta$ evaluated at $\theta_1 = \hat{\theta}_1$ and $\theta_2 = 0$) takes the form

$$T_S = [0, U_2(\theta)] \begin{bmatrix} I_{f11} & I_{f12} \\ I_{f21} & I_{f22} \end{bmatrix}^{-1} \begin{bmatrix} 0 \\ U_2(\theta) \end{bmatrix}.$$

$$= U_2(\theta)^T \left(I_{f22} - I_{f21}I_{f11}^{-1}I_{f12}\right)^{-1} U_2(\theta) \tag{5.86}$$

Under H_0 and a correctly specified likelihood, $T_S \overset{d}{\to} \chi^2_{r_2}$.

Generalized Score Test

Frequently, the problem arises that the likelihood of the current model is mis-specified and accordingly the statistical inference might be incorrect. For example, overdispersion frequently occurs in the case of count data where a Poisson model is assumed. Thus, it is desirable to allow for model misspecification. For that matter, see, for example, Boos (1992) or Breslow (1990), who suggest the use of gener-alized score tests. As before the key element is given by $E(U) = 0$ and $\hat{\theta}$, which solves $U(\hat{\theta}) = 0$. This result not only applies to maximum likelihood estimation, but also to least-squares or generalized estimating equations.

The following ideas on generalized score tests are asymptotic results based on Taylor series expansions. The asymptotic distribution of $\hat{\theta}$ is given by the Taylor series expansion

$$0 = U(\hat{\theta}) = S(\theta) + \frac{\partial U(\theta)}{\partial \theta}(\hat{\theta} - \theta) + o_p(1), \tag{5.87}$$

where $o_p(1)$ denotes a quantity that converges to 0 in probability. From results of Iganaki (1973), the estimator $\hat{\theta}$ is asymptotically normal and consistent with variance

$$\mathrm{var}\,(\hat{\theta} - \theta) = I_g^{-1} D_g I_g^{-1}, \tag{5.88}$$

$$I_g = \lim_{n \to \infty} \left[-E \frac{\partial U(\theta)}{\partial \theta} \right], \tag{5.89}$$

$$(D_g)_{r_1 r_2} = \lim_{n \to \infty} \left[\frac{1}{n} \sum_{i=1}^n E\left(\frac{\partial \ell}{\partial \theta_{r_1}} \frac{\partial \ell}{\partial \theta_{r_2}}\right) \right]. \tag{5.90}$$

Then $\hat{\theta}$ has variance covariance matrix $V_g = I_g^{-1} D_g I_g^{-1}$. This is a familiar result from robust statistics (Huber 1967), generalized estimating equations (Liang and Zeger 1986), or misspecified maximum likelihood estimation; see, for example, White

(1982). Instead of the matrices of expectations I_g and D_g, the empirical covariance matrix is frequently used:

$$V_Y = I_Y^{-1} D_Y I_Y^{-1}, \tag{5.91}$$

where I_Y is the observed information and D_Y (the empirical version of D_g) is given by

$$D_Y = \sum_{i=1}^{n} u_i(\theta) u_i(\theta)^{\mathrm{T}}, \tag{5.92}$$

where u_i is the ith contribution to the score $U(\theta)$.

As an example consider a linear model with dependent variable Y: $E(Y) = X\beta$. Standard likelihood inference leads to an estimate for the variance $I_Y = \hat{\sigma}^2 (X^{\mathrm{T}} X)$. The score is given by $U = \frac{1}{\hat{\sigma}^2}(y - X\hat{\beta})X$. Applying (5.91) leads to the variance estimate $V_Y = (X^{\mathrm{T}} X)^{-1} X^{\mathrm{T}} R X (X^{\mathrm{T}} X)^{-1}$, where R are the squared residuals. Note that if R is replaced by $R = I\hat{\sigma}^2$, the identity matrix times the average residuals squared, the usual variance estimate is obtained. In other words, if the variance is correctly specified, (5.91) gives the usual variance estimate.

Now, returning to the score test on subvectors, we expand U_1 and U_2 by a Taylor series. If $\hat{\theta}_1$ is the maximum likelihood estimator for the restricted model and $\theta = (\theta_1^{\mathrm{T}}, \theta_2^{\mathrm{T}})$ for any arbitrary $\theta_2 \in \mathbb{R}^{r_2}$ model, we get

$$0 = U_1(\hat{\theta}) = U_1(\theta) + \frac{\partial U_1}{\partial \theta_1}(\hat{\theta}_1 - \theta_1) + o_p(1) \Leftrightarrow$$

$$(\hat{\theta}_1 - \theta_1) \approx \left[\frac{\partial U_1}{\partial \theta_1}\right]^{-1} U_1(\theta), \tag{5.93}$$

and for U_2 we get

$$U_2(\hat{\theta}) = U_2(\theta) + \frac{\partial U_2}{\partial \theta_1}(\hat{\theta}_1 - \theta_1) + o_p(1) \Leftrightarrow \tag{5.94}$$

$$U_2(\hat{\theta}) = U_2(\theta) - \frac{\partial U_2}{\partial \theta_1}\left[\frac{\partial U_1}{\partial \theta_1}\right]^{-1} U_1(\theta). \tag{5.95}$$

This can be written as

$$U_2(\hat{\theta}) = \left[I_{r_2}, -I_{g21} I_{g11}^{-1}\right] \begin{bmatrix} U_2 \\ U_1 \end{bmatrix}. \tag{5.96}$$

Since the variance of the score $\mathrm{var}(U) = E(U^{\mathrm{T}} U)$, it follows that the variance of (5.96) is given by

$$V_{\mathrm{GS}} = \left[I_r, -I_{g21} I_{g11}^{-1}\right] D_g \left[I_r, -I_{g21} I_{g11}^{-1}\right]^{\mathrm{T}} \tag{5.97}$$

$$= D_{g22} - I_{g21} I_{g11}^{-1} D_{g21}^{\mathrm{T}} - D_{g21} I_{g11}^{-1} I_{g21}^{\mathrm{T}} + I_{g21} I_{g11}^{-1} D_{g11} I_{g11}^{-1} I_{g21}^{\mathrm{T}}. \tag{5.98}$$

Replacing I_g and D_g by the observed quantities leads again to the empirical score test.

Chapter 6
Modeling Heterogeneity in Psychophysiology

6.1 The Electroencephalogram

Neuronal population activity in the human cortex generates electric fields which are measurable by placing electrodes at the skull. The electroencephalography (EEG) electrodes are fixed with paste on the scalp and electrical activity is recorded on paper or is stored digitally. The voltage of EEG is low and is measured in tens of microvolts. Traditional EEG systems use 20 electrodes which are fixed to the scalp using paste. The location of the electrodes on the scalp often follows the 10-20 system in order to provide a standardized way to place the electrodes. For example, the locations F_z, C_z and P_z are obtained by subdividing the distance between nasion and inion in pieces of 10 or 20%, which led to the name of the 10-20 system.

Figure 6.1 shows a schematic representation of the 10-20 system with standard electrode names and positions. Obviously there is only limited spatial information, but EEG offers high temporal resolution. Owing to the low spatial resolution, EEG is no longer the only method which provides information on the functioning of the brain. It has to be contrasted with methods such as positron emission tomography and functional magnetic resonance imaging. EEG is totally noninvasive (in contrast to positron emission tomography) and offers a very high temporal resolution on the order of milliseconds. Thus, the major advantage of EEG is its relative ease of application together with low cost of data acquisition.

6.1.1 Digitization

The electroencephalogram is nowadays almost always recorded and stored electronically. The analogue signals are digitized with a sampling rate v of 200 Hz or more on modern machines. This implies a sampling interval $\Delta t = 1/v = 0.005$ s. Thus, at a sampling rate of 200 Hz, we record discrete signals $x_i(t)$, $t = 0, \ldots, N-1$, where an epoch of T seconds leads to $N = T/\Delta t$ discrete values. This is recorded

P. Schlattmann, *Medical Applications of Finite Mixture Models*,
Statistics for Biology and Health, DOI: 10.1007/978-3-540-68651-4_6,
© Springer-Verlag Berlin Hiedelberg 2009

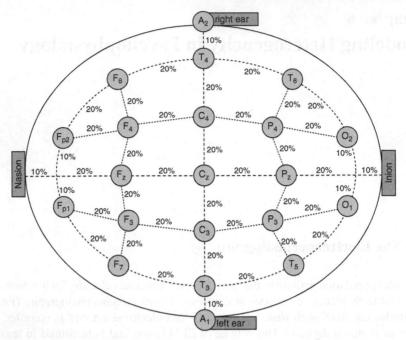

Fig. 6.1 Standard electroencephalography (EEG) electrode locations

at $l = 1,\ldots,L$ electrode positions. Thus, performing EEG studies leads to a massive amount of data. Suppose that a study with 20 patients and 20 controls is conducted, where for each subject 10 min of EEG data with a sampling rate of 200 MHz are recorded at 20 electrode positions. This leads to 96 million data points! Thus, suitable methods for data reduction have to be found which provide meaningful information for each subject.

An initial useful representation of EEG data is to present a plot of the time series of the EEG recordings at each electrode. A time series plot of an example electroencephalogram according to the 10-20 system with a recording length of 3 s is shown in Fig. 6.2.

6.2 Modeling Spatial Heterogeneity Using Generalized Linear Mixed Models

6.2.1 The Periodogram and its Distributional Properties

One frequently used method of data reduction in the EEG literature is the transformation of the EEG time series from the time domain into the frequency domain. This is achieved by considering an observed time series as the realization of a stationary

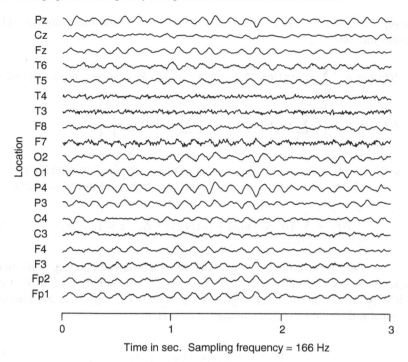

Fig. 6.2 Three seconds of EEG recording of a healthy male individual

random process $Y(t), t = 1, \ldots, n$ with spectral density $f(\omega)$ which needs to be estimated from the data. Note that the assumption of stationarity is not necessarily true for EEG data. As a result, mainly short time intervals are considered for an analysis in the frequency domain. The literature on spectral analysis is extensive. A text from a biostatistical point of view is the monograph by Diggle (1990). Other accessible texts are the monographs by Bloomfield (2000), Schlittgen and Streitberg (2001), and Chatfield (2004). The spectrum of a stationary process $\{Y\}$ is defined as the discrete Fourier transform of its autocovariance function. If $\gamma_k = \text{Cov}\{Y_t, Y_{t-k}\}$ denotes the autocovariance function, then its Fourier transform is given by

$$f(\omega) = \sum_{-\infty}^{\infty} \gamma_k \exp(-ik\omega), \quad (0 < \omega < \pi). \tag{6.1}$$

Here ω denotes the frequency and $\exp(i\omega k)$ is defined as the exponential function based on complex numbers:

$$e^{i\omega} = \cos(\omega k) + i\sin(\omega k), \tag{6.2}$$

where $\cos(\omega k)$ is the real part and $i\sin(\omega k)$ is the imaginary part, with imaginary unit i. The imaginary unit has the property $i^2 = -1$. One possible estimator for $f(\omega)$ is the periodogram ordinate $I(\omega)$. Considering only *Fourier frequencies*, i.e., of the form $\omega_j = 2\pi j/n$ for a positive integer $j < n/2$ leads to the following equivalent formulae for $I(\omega)$:

$$I(\omega_j) = n^{-1} \sum_{t=1}^{n} x_t \exp(i\omega_j t)^2, \quad j = 1,\ldots,M, \quad M = \frac{n-1}{2}, \quad \omega_j = 2\pi j/n \quad (6.3)$$

$$I(\omega_j) = n^{-1} \left[\left(\sum_{t=1}^{n} x_t \cos(\omega_j t) \right)^2 + \left(\sum_{t=1}^{n} x_t \sin(\omega_j t) \right)^2 \right].$$

The periodogram ordinates $I(\omega_j)$ may be obtained by decomposing the time series $y(t)$ into harmonic components, each with two degrees of freedom. That is,

$$y(t) = \sum_{j=1}^{M} (\alpha_j \cos(\omega_j t) + \beta_j(\omega_j t)) + \varepsilon_i, \quad t = 1,\ldots,n, \quad (6.4)$$

where ε is a white noise sequence and each ω_j is a Fourier frequency. This model is linear in the coefficients α_j and β_j and estimation may simply be done by treating this task as a multiple linear regression problem. The regressors are mutually orthogonal and thus the explicit solutions are given by

$$\hat{\alpha}_j = 2 \left(\sum_{i=1}^{n} y_i \cos(\omega_j t) \right) / n, \quad (6.5)$$

$$\hat{\beta}_j = 2 \left(\sum_{i=1}^{n} y_i \sin(\omega_j t) \right) / n. \quad (6.6)$$

Note that the periodogram is usually calculated using a fast Fourier transform algorithm (Cooley and Tukey 1965). These algorithms are available in statistical packages such as R and SAS. The fast Fourier transform is much faster than direct calculation and from it the periodogram is available at the fundamental frequencies ω_j, $2\pi j/n$, $0 \leq j \leq M = n/2$.

As seen in Fig. 6.3, the raw periodogram is too variable to be useful visually and according to some authors (Gasser and Molinari 1996) it is also not useful quantitatively. The kernel estimated spectrum shows a peak structure, with a strong alpha rhythm at about 8 Hz. In the EEG literature many derivatives of the raw periodogram are used for further analysis. Among these are peak frequencies, some measures of broadness of the peak, and a parameter of power obtained by summing the power of the peak. Based on the periodogram, the most frequently used spectral power parameters are depicted in Fig. 6.3 and are listed in Table 6.1. The categorization of the spectrum into categories, i.e., frequency bands, is mostly based on clinical convention; however, attempts to find categorization-based quantitative methods by means of a factor analysis lead to similar categories (Herrmann et al. 1978). Frequently, data analysis is restricted to certain bands such as the alpha band. Clearly, this results in a loss of information. Thus, we propose and develop model-based approaches which make use of the entire information provided by the periodogram.

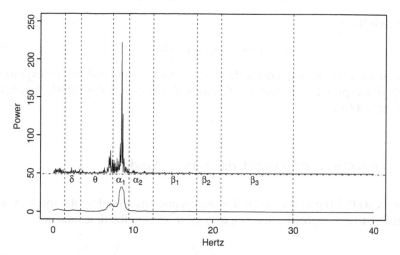

Fig. 6.3 Raw periodogram activity of a healthy control at left occipital location O_1 (*upper trace*). The *lower trace* is a kernel estimated spectrum. *Dashed vertical lines* denote boundaries of conventional frequency bands to obtain band power parameters (sum of power in bands)

Table 6.1 Clinical electroencephalography frequency bands

Frequency (Hz)	Name	State of mind
0–3.5	Delta	Coma, deep sleep
4–8	Theta	Sleep, relaxation
8–13	Alpha	Relaxed wakefulness
14–40	Beta	Agitated wakefulness

The periodogram evaluated at the Fourier frequencies is readily interpretable and has nice statistical properties such as that the periodogram ordinate $I(\omega_j)$ may be interpreted as the sum of squares with two degrees of freedom attributable to the harmonic regression function:

$$\mu_j(t) = \alpha_j \cos(\omega_j t) + \beta_j \sin(\omega_j t), \quad t = 1, \ldots, n. \qquad (6.7)$$

The periodogram ordinate at the jth Fourier frequency

$$I(\omega_j) = \frac{n}{4(\alpha_j^2 + \beta_j^2)}, \quad j = 1, \ldots, 2\pi j/n,$$

is therefore half of the sum of squares due to regression on the pair of sinusoids with that frequency.

The asymptotic distribution theory of the periodogram ordinates $I(\omega_j)$ is remarkably simple. For a stationary process the distributional properties may be summarized by the following. Asymptotically in n, for each $j = 1, \ldots, n$ we have

$$I(\omega_j) \sim \exp[f(\omega_j, \theta)], \quad \omega_j = 2\pi, \qquad (6.8)$$

and for each $i \neq j$

$$I(\omega_i) \text{ and } I(\omega_j) \text{ are independent.} \tag{6.9}$$

Thus, at the Fourier frequencies the periodogram simply follows an exponential distribution $\exp(\cdot)$. Details and proofs may be found in Priestley (1991, Sect. 6.1) or Brillinger (2001).

6.3 Connection to Generalized Linear Models

Bloomfield (1973) proposed the following exponential model for the spectrum as an alternative to autoregressive moving average models in the time domain:

$$f(\omega, \theta) = \exp\left(2 \sum_{k=0}^{m} \beta_k \cos(k\omega) \right). \tag{6.10}$$

As a result of the distributional properties of the periodogram ordinates in (6.8) and (6.9), time series models based on the spectrum fall into the generalized linear models framework as described in Sect. 4.6.1 on page 87. This idea in connection with the spectrum of scalar time series was pioneered by Cameron and Turner (1987). Thus, fitting a generalized linear regression model to the EEG data, one finds that the error distribution of the dependent variable $I(\omega_j)$ is given by the exponential or more generally the gamma distribution. The link function $g(\cdot)$ is the logarithmic link and the linear predictor is given by the term $\eta = X\theta$. Here θ is the vector of m unknown regression coefficients and X is the design matrix as described in (6.11):

$$\text{Design matrix} \quad X: \quad x_{jk} = 2\cos(k\omega_j) \quad k = 0, \ldots m, \tag{6.11}$$

$$\theta = (\beta_0, \beta_1, \ldots, \beta_m)^T, \tag{6.12}$$

$$\eta = X\theta, \tag{6.13}$$

$$g(\mu_j) = \eta_j. \tag{6.14}$$

Estimation of the model's parameters is usually done using maximum likelihood. The likelihood to be maximized is given by

$$L(I(\omega_1, \theta), \ldots, I(\omega_M, \theta)) = \prod_{i=1}^{M} f(\omega_j, \theta) \exp\left[-f(\omega_j, \theta)I(\omega_j)\right].$$

The corresponding log likelihood function is given by

$$\ell(\theta) = \sum_{j=1}^{M} X_j \theta - f(\omega_j, \theta)I(\omega_j),$$

$$\ell(\theta) = \sum_{j=1}^{M} \eta_j - \exp(\eta_j)I(\omega_j). \tag{6.15}$$

This log likelihood can be maximized using the iterative weighted least squares algorithm (Algorithm 4.6.1) on page 90 since the exponential distribution belongs to the exponential family. This is shown in Example 4.6 on page 88.

As for other generalized linear models, parameter estimates may be obtained using standard software packages such as R, SAS, and STATA. Figure 6.4 shows the periodogram ordinates $I(\omega_j)$ together with a fitted regression line for each electrode b to the 10-20 system based on a generalized linear model based on the EEG time series displayed in Fig. 6.2. The number of regression parameters m is set to 6. Thus, in terms of data reduction this procedure does not offer a real advantage over classical methods based on periodogram ordinates since 144 parameters need to be estimated from the data.

6.3.1 Covariate-Adjusted Finite Mixture Models for the EEG Data

To reduce the number of parameters which need to be estimated and to address spatial variability between electrodes a covariate-adjusted finite mixture model can be applied to the data. This is quite similar to the applications in other contexts because a discrete latent distribution for the random effects P is assumed. The only difference is that is the periodogram ordinates are assumed to follow an exponential distribution. The mixing distribution is given by

$$P = \begin{bmatrix} \theta_1 & \cdots & \theta_q \\ p_1 & \cdots & p_q \end{bmatrix}. \tag{6.16}$$

Again, the parameters $\theta_1, \ldots, \theta_q$ are no longer scalar quantities but vectors, e.g.,

$$\theta_1 = (\beta_{01}, \beta_{11}, \ldots, \beta_{m1}), \tag{6.17}$$

where m denotes the number of covariates in the model. Again, in contrast to the homogenous case we have the same type of density $f(\cdot)$ for each subpopulation but a different parameter vector θ_j in subpopulation $j = 1, \ldots, q$.

Similar to the development in Sect. 4.7 where the latent distribution considers a mixture of concentration–time curves and a mixture of individual concentration curves is considered, here a mixture of time series per electrode is analyzed. If we assume conditional independence for each electrode, the density $f(\cdot)$ is given by the product of the exponential densities of that electrode. That is, the mixture distribution for the ith electrode is given by $I_i(\omega)$:

$$f(I_i(\omega), P) \sim p_1 f(I_i(\omega), \theta_1) + \cdots + p_k f(I_i(\omega), \theta_q) \quad q \quad \text{components,}$$

$$f(I_i(\omega), \theta_r) = \prod_j^{M_i} \exp(I(\omega_j, \exp(\eta_{ij})) \quad M_i \quad \text{frequencies.}$$

In contrast to the pooled model for all electrodes shown in Fig. 6.5, a covariate-adjusted mixture model does provide a satisfactory fit to the periodogram ordinates (Fig. 6.6). This framework can be easily extended to many individuals and thus may be used for model-based analysis of EEG data.

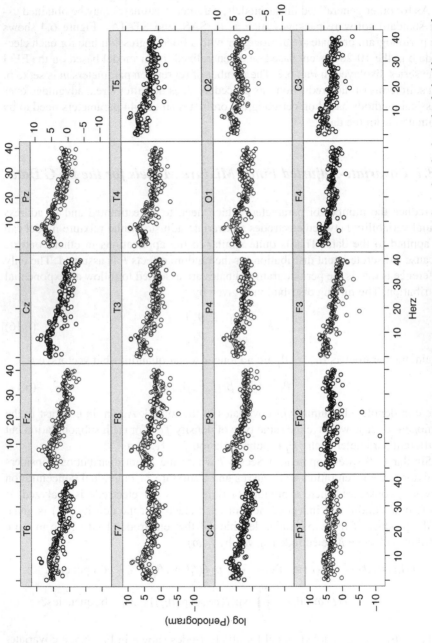

Fig. 6.4 Periodogram ordinates $I(\omega)$ and fitted regression line derived by a generalized linear model for each scalp electrode of a healthy control

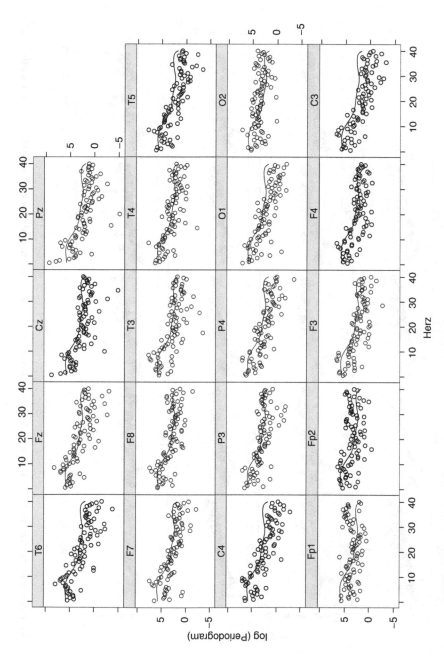

Fig. 6.5 Periodogram ordinates $I(\omega)$ and fitted regression lines derived by a pooled generalized linear model for scalp electrodes of a healthy control

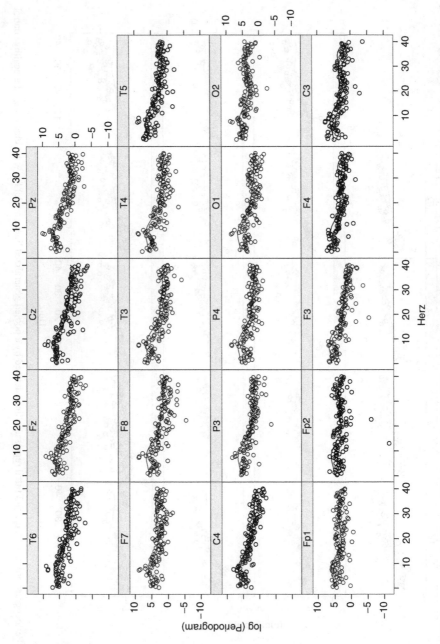

Fig. 6.6 Periodogram ordinates $I(\omega)$ and fitted regression lines fit by a covariate-adjusted mixture model for each scalp electrode of a healthy control

Chapter 7
Investigating and Analyzing Heterogeneity in Meta-analysis

7.1 Introduction

Meta-analysis may be defined as (Glass 1976):

> The statistical analysis of a large collection of analysis results for the purpose if integrating these findings.

This has to be contrasted with *primary research*, which denotes the direct investigation of human or animal data. Providing a report of primary research using statistical methodology and analysis is often called a quantitative review in contrast to a narrative review. In principle, a meta-analysis provides the same methodological rigor to a literature review that is required for primary research.

Meta-analysis has become popular in many areas of medical and social sciences. It has been estimated by Egger et al. (1998) that from articles retrieved by MEDLINE with the medical subject heading (MeSH) term "meta-analysis" some 33% reported results of a meta-analysis from randomized clinical trials and nearly the same proportion (27%) were from observational studies, including 12% papers in which the cause of a disease was investigated. The remaining papers include methodological publications or review articles. Reasons for the popularity of meta-analyses are the growing amount of information in the scientific literature and the need for timely decisions for risk assessment or in public health. Often a meta-analysis tries to combine the evidence of many independent studies and thus aims to provide a quantitative review of the literature. Methods for meta-analyses to summarize or synthesize evidence from randomized controlled clinical trials have been continuously developed. These methods are now summarized in several textbooks; see, for example, Sutton et al. (2000) and Whitehead (2001) and the handbook by Egger et al. (2001). A general overview of recent developments in statistical methods for meta-analysis may be found in the review by Sutton and Higgins (2008). In epidemiology a recent review on meta-analysis may be found in the article by Blettner and Schlattmann (2007) published in the *Handbook of Epidemiology* (Ahrens and Pigeot 2007). Dickersin (2002) argued that statistical methods for meta-analyses of

P. Schlattmann, *Medical Applications of Finite Mixture Models*,
Statistics for Biology and Health, DOI: 10.1007/978-3-540-68651-4_7,
© Springer-Verlag Berlin Hiedelberg 2009

epidemiologic studies still lag behind in comparison with the progress that has been made for randomized clinical trials. The use of meta-analyses for epidemiologic research resulted in many controversial discussions; see for, example, Blettner et al. (1999), Berlin (1995), Greenland (1994), Feinstein (1995), Olkin (1994), Shapiro (1994a,b), and Weed (1997) for a detailed overview of the arguments. The most prominent arguments against meta-analyses are the fundamental issues of confounding, selection bias, as well as the large variety and heterogeneity of study designs and data collection procedures in epidemiologic research. Despite these controversies, results from meta-analyses are often cited and used for decisions. They are often seen as the fundamentals for risk assessment. They are also performed to summarize the current state of knowledge often prior to designing new studies.

7.1.1 Different Types of Overviews

Approaches for summarizing evidence include four different types of overviews:

1. Traditional narrative reviews that provide a qualitative but not a quantitative assessment of published results. Methods and guidelines for reviews have been published (Weed 1997).
2. Meta-analyses from the literature which are generally performed using freely available publications without the need of cooperation and without agreement of the authors from the original studies. They are comparable to a narrative review in many respects but include quantitative estimate(s) of the effect of interest. One example is a meta-analysis by Zeeger et al. (2003) of studies investigating some familial clustering of prostate cancer. A meta-analysis on the association between Parkinson disease, smoking, and family history was recently published in Allam et al. (2003).
3. Meta-analyses with individual patient data in which individual data from published and sometimes also unpublished studies are reanalyzed. Often, there is close cooperation between the researcher performing the meta-analysis and the investigators of the individual studies. The new analysis may include specific inclusion criteria for patients and controls, new definition of the exposure and confounder variables, and new statistical modeling. This reanalysis may overcome some but not all of the problems of meta-analyses of published data (Blettner et al. 1999). They have been performed in epidemiologic research for many years. One of the largest investigations of this form was an investigation on breast cancer and oral contraceptive use, where data from 54 case-control studies were pooled and reanalyzed (Breast Cancer 1996). A further international collaboration led by Lubin et al. (1995) was set up to reanalyze data from 11 large cohort studies on lung cancer and radon among uranium miners. The reanalysis allowed a refined dose-response analysis and provided data for radiation protection issues. Pooled reanalyses are mostly performed by combining data from studies of the same type only. For example, Hung et al. (2003) reanalyzed data from all case-control studies in which the role of genetic polymorphisms for lung cancer

in nonsmokers were investigated. The role of diet for lung cancer was recently reviewed by Smith-Warner et al. (2002) in a qualitative and quantitative way by combining cohort studies. An overview of methodological aspects for a pooled analysis of data from cohort studies was published in Bennett (2003). Currently, methods are under development which allow one to combine individual and aggregate data. See, for example, the work by Riley et al. (2007) or Sutton et al. (2008) .

4. Prospectively planned pooled meta-analyses of several studies in which pooling is already a part of the protocol. Data collection procedures and definitions of variables are standardized as far as possible for the individual studies. The statistical analysis has many similarities with the meta-analysis based on individual data. A major difference, however, is that joint planning of the data collection and analysis increases the homogeneity of the data sets included. However, in contrast to multicenter randomized clinical trials, important heterogeneity between the study centers may still exist. This heterogeneity may arise from differences in populations, in the relevant confounding variables (e.g., race may only be a confounder in some centers), and potential differences in ascertainment of controls.

7.2 Basic Statistical Analysis

The statistical analysis of aggregated data from published studies was first developed in the fields of psychology and education (Glass 1977; Smith and Glass 1977). Since the mid-1980s these methods have been adopted in medicine primarily for randomized clinical trials and are also used for epidemiologic data. We will give a brief outline of some issues of the analysis using an example based on a meta-analysis performed by Sillero-Arenas et al. (1992). This study was one of the first meta-analyses which tried to summarize quantitatively the association between hormone replacement therapy (HRT) and breast cancer in women. Sillero-Arenas et al. based their meta-analysis on 23 case-control studies and 13 cohort studies. The data extracted from the paper by Sillero-Arenas et al. are displayed in Table 7.1. This table shows the study number and the logarithm of the odds ratio (OR) or relative risk, the last two denoted as log (OR) for brevity. Additionally the corresponding estimate of variance on the log scale and the covariate study type is listed, where a case-control study has the value 0 and a cohort study has the value 1.

7.2.1 Single Study Results

A first step of the statistical analysis is the description of the characteristics and the results of each study. Tabulations and simple graphical methods should be employed to visualize the results of the single studies. Plotting the ORs and their confidence intervals (so-called forest plot) is a simple way to spot obvious differences between

Table 7.1 Data on hormone replacement therapy and breast cancer extracted from Sillero-Arenas et al. (1992). Here 0 denotes a case-control study and 1 a cohort study

Study	log(OR)	Variance	Type
1	0.10436	0.299111	0
2	−0.03046	0.121392	0
3	0.76547	0.319547	0
4	−0.19845	0.025400	0
5	−0.10536	0.025041	0
6	−0.11653	0.040469	0
7	0.09531	0.026399	0
8	0.26236	0.017918	0
9	−0.26136	0.020901	0
10	0.45742	0.035877	0
11	−0.59784	0.076356	0
12	−0.35667	0.186879	0
13	−0.10536	0.089935	0
14	−0.31471	0.013772	0
15	−0.10536	0.089935	0
16	0.02956	0.004738	0
17	0.60977	0.035781	0
18	−0.30111	0.036069	0
19	0.01980	0.024611	0
20	0.00000	0.002890	0
21	−0.04082	0.015863	0
22	0.02956	0.067069	0
23	0.18232	0.010677	0
24	0.26236	0.017918	1
25	0.32208	0.073896	1
26	0.67803	0.489415	1
27	−0.96758	0.194768	1
28	0.91629	0.051846	1
29	0.32208	0.110179	1
30	−0.13943	0.086173	1
31	−0.47804	0.103522	1
32	0.16551	0.004152	1
33	0.46373	0.023150	1
34	−0.52763	0.050384	1
35	0.10436	0.003407	1
36	0.55389	0.054740	1

OR odds ratio

the study results. Figure 7.1 shows a forest plot of 36 studies investigating the association of HRT and breast cancer in women.

An alternative way to display the individual study's results graphically is a bubble plot, where the size of the bubble is inversely proportional to the study-specific variance. An example is shown in Fig. 7.2

Looking at the plots in Figs. 7.1 and 7.2, we see there is a high variability of effects between studies. Later we will describe how to account for heterogeneity of studies quantitatively.

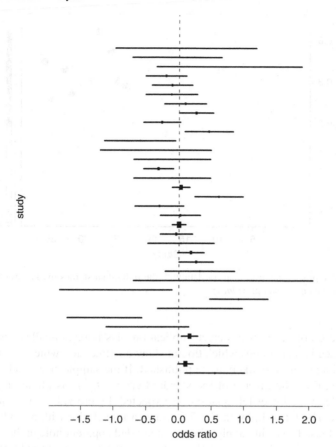

Fig. 7.1 Forest plot of the breast cancer data

7.2.2 Publication Bias

An important problem of meta-analysis is publication bias. This bias has received a lot of attention particularly in the area of clinical trials. Publication bias occurs when studies that have nonsignificant or negative results are published less frequently than studies with positive results. For randomized clinical trials, it has been shown that even with a computer-aided literature search not all of the relevant studies will be identified (Dickersin et al. 1994). For epidemiologic observational studies additional problems exist, because often a large number of variables will be collected in questionnaires as potential confounders. If one or several of these potential confounders yield significant or important results, they may be published in additional papers, which have often not been planned in advance. In general, publication bias yields a nonnegligible overestimation of the risk estimate. As a result, prior to further statistical analyses, publication bias should be investigated.

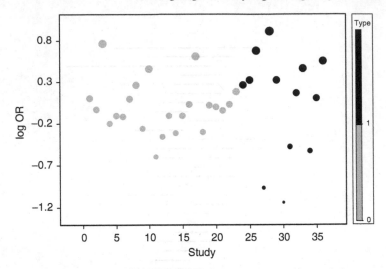

Fig. 7.2 Bubble plot of the breast cancer data with the individual studies marked as case-control studies (*gray*) and cohort studies (*black*)

A simple graphical tool to detect publication bias is the so-called funnel plot. The basic idea is that studies which do not show an effect and which are not statistically significant are less likely to be published. If the sample size, or alternatively the precision (i.e., the inverse of the standard error (σ_i^{-1})), is plotted against the effect, a hole in the lower-left quadrant is expected. Figure 7.3 shows examples of funnel plots. The left subplot in Fig. 7.3 shows a funnel plot with no indication of publication bias. The right subplot shows a so-called apparent hole in the lower-left corner. In the case of the right subplot in Fig. 7.3 the presence of publication bias would be assumed. Figure 7.4 shows a funnel plot for the breast cancer data, where no apparent hole in the lower-left corner is present. Thus, no publication bias would be assumed.

For a quantitative investigation of publication bias, several methods are available. These may be based on statistical tests; see, for example, Begg and Mazumdar (1994) or Schwarzer et al. (2002). A recent simulation study performed by Macaskill et al. (2001) favored the use of regression methods. The basic idea is to regress the estimated effect sizes $\hat{\theta}_i$ directly on the sample size or the inverse variance σ_i^{-2} as a predictor. An alternative idea is to use Egger's regression test (Egger et al. 1997), which uses standardized study-specific effects as a dependent variable and the corresponding precision as an independent variable. Simulation studies by Macaskill et al. (2001) and by Peters et al. (2006) have indicated that the method proposed by Macaskill is superior to Egger's method. Thus, our analysis is restricted to the method of Macaskill, which leads to the following regression model :

$$\hat{\theta}_i = \alpha + \beta \frac{1}{\hat{\sigma}_i^2} + \varepsilon_i, \qquad i = 1, \ldots, k, \quad \varepsilon_i \sim N(0, \sigma_i^2). \tag{7.1}$$

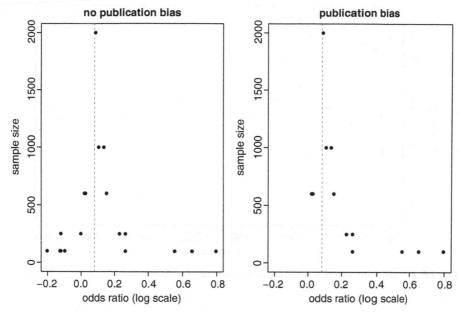

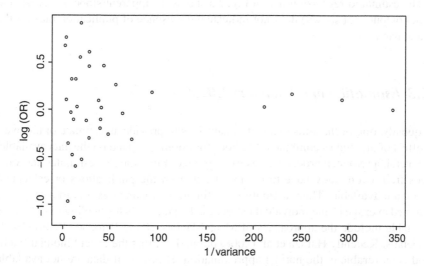

Fig. 7.3 Examples of funnel plots based on simulated data with (*right*) and without (*left*) publication bias present. The *dotted line* shows the true effect

Fig. 7.4 Funnel plot of the breast cancer data

Here, the number of studies to be pooled is denoted by k. Note that we used the inverse variance as a surrogate for the sample size n_i of the ith study. In this model it is assumed that the estimated treatment effects are independently normally distributed. With no publication bias present the regression line should be parallel to the x-axis, i.e., the slope should be zero. A nonzero slope would suggest an association between

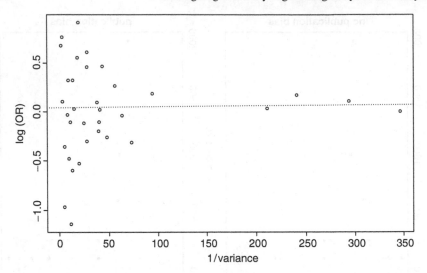

Fig. 7.5 Funnel regression plot of the breast cancer data

sample size or inverse variance and effect size, possibly due to publication bias. Additionally the observations are weighted by the inverse variance.

The estimated regression line in Fig. 7.5 shows no apparent slope. Likewise, the model output (not shown) does not indicate the presence of publication bias for the data at hand.

7.2.3 Estimation of a Summary Effect

Frequently, one of the aims of a meta-analysis is to provide an estimate of the overall effect of all studies combined. Methods for pooling depend on the data available. In general, a two-step procedure has to be applied. First, the risk estimates and variances from each study have to be abstracted from the publications or calculated if data are available. Then, a combined estimate is obtained as a (variance-based) weighted average of the individual estimates. The methods for pooling based on the 2×2 table include the approaches of Mantel-Haenszel and Peto; see Pettiti (1994) for details. Recently Hamza et al. (2008) pointed out that the exact binomial likelihood is preferable to the normal approximation. However, if data are not available in a 2×2 table, but are available as an estimate from a more complex model (such as an adjusted relative risk estimate), the Woolf approach can be adopted using the estimates and their (published or calculated) variance resulting from the regression model. In the following it will be shown how a summary effect $\hat{\theta}$ can be obtained as a weighted average of the log (ORs) $\hat{\theta}_i$ of the individual studies. The weights w_i are given by the inverse of the study-specific variance estimates $\hat{\sigma}_i^2$. Note that the study-specific variances are assumed to be fixed and known although they are estimates.

As a result, the uncertainty associated with the estimation of σ_i^2 is ignored. Thus, in the following the σ_i are treated as constants and the "hat" notation is omitted.

Estimation of the summary effect θ may be done using maximum likelihood. Assuming a normal distribution for the individual study leads to the following likelihood:

$$L(\theta) = \prod_{i=1}^{k} \frac{1}{\sqrt{2\pi\sigma_i^2}} \exp\left[-\frac{(\hat{\theta}_i - \theta)^2}{2\sigma_i^2}\right] \qquad i = 1,\ldots,k. \qquad (7.2)$$

More convenient is the log likelihood:

$$\ell(\theta) = \sum_{i=1}^{k}\left[-\log\left(\sqrt{2\pi\sigma_i^2}\right) - \frac{(\hat{\theta}_i - \theta)^2}{2\sigma_i^2}\right]. \qquad (7.3)$$

The *score* is given by taking the first derivative of the log likelihood function:

$$\ell'(\theta) = \frac{d\ell(\theta)}{d\theta} = \sum_{i=1}^{k} \frac{(\hat{\theta}_i - \theta)}{\sigma_i^2}. \qquad (7.4)$$

This leads to the *score equation*:

$$\ell'(\theta) = 0 \quad \text{or} \quad \sum_{i=1}^{k} \frac{\hat{\theta}_i}{\sigma_i^2} = \theta \sum_{i=1}^{k} \frac{1}{\sigma_i^2}. \qquad (7.5)$$

The estimate of the summary effect of all studies is then given by

$$\hat{\theta} = \frac{\sum_{i=1}^{k} w_i \hat{\theta}_i}{\sum_{i=1}^{k} w_i}, \qquad w_i = \frac{1}{\sigma_i^2}.$$

Using the expected Fisher information, the variance is

$$I(\theta) = E\left[-\frac{d^2\ell(\theta)}{d\theta^2}\right]$$

$$= E\left[-\sum_{i=1}^{n} \frac{-1}{\sigma_i^2}\right] = \sum_{i=1}^{k} \frac{1}{\sigma_i^2},$$

$$\text{var}(\hat{\theta}) = \frac{1}{\sum_{i=1}^{k} \frac{1}{\sigma_i^2}}. \qquad (7.6)$$

Applying this approach to the HRT data leads to a pooled risk estimate of 0.065598 with an estimated variance of 0.00051. Transforming this back to the original scale leads to an OR of 1.058 with a 95% confidence interval of 1.012–1.11. Thus, we would conclude from combining all studies that there is a small harmful effect of HRT.

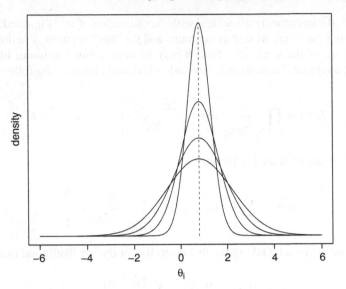

Fig. 7.6 Fixed effects model: common effect with different study variances

The major assumption here is that of a fixed effects model, i.e., it is assumed that the underlying true exposure effect in each study is the same. The overall variation and, therefore, the confidence intervals will reflect only the random variation within each study but not any potential heterogeneity between the studies. Figure 7.6 displays this idea. Whether pooling of the data is appropriate should be decided after investigating the heterogeneity of the study results. If the results vary substantially, no pooled estimator should be presented or only estimators for selected subgroups should be calculated (e.g., combining results from case-control studies only).

7.3 Analysis of Heterogeneity

The previous remark notwithstanding, as Senn (2007) points out a fixed effect meta-analysis is always valuable, since it tests the null hypothesis that, e.g., treatments were identical in all trials. If the null hypothesis is rejected, then the alternative may be asserted that at least one treatment differs. Thus, the investigation of heterogeneity between the different studies is a main task in each review or meta-analysis (Thompson 1994). For the quantitative assessment of heterogeneity, several statistical tests are available (Paul and Donner 1989; Pettiti 1994). A simple test for heterogeneity is based on the following test statistic

$$\chi^2_{\text{het}} = \sum_{i=1}^{k} \frac{(\hat{\theta} - \hat{\theta}_i)^2}{\sigma_i^2} \sim \chi^2_{k-1}, \tag{7.7}$$

which under the null hypothesis of homogeneity follows a χ^2 distribution with $k-1$ degrees of freedom. Hence, the null hypothesis is rejected if χ^2_{het} exceeds the $1-\alpha$ quantile of χ^2_{k-1} denoted as $\chi^2_{k-1,1-\alpha}$. For the data at hand we clearly conclude that there is heterogeneity present ($\chi^2_{\text{het}} = 116.076$, 35 degrees of freedom, $p = 0.0000$). Thus, using a combined estimate is at least questionable. Pooling the individual studies and performing this test can be done with any statistical package capable of weighted least squares regression.

However, this test only carries information about the presence versus the absence of heterogeneity, and it does not report on the extent of such heterogeneity. As a result, the I^2 index has been proposed to quantify the degree of heterogeneity:

$$I^2 = \max\left(0, \frac{\chi^2_{\text{het}} - \text{df}}{\chi^2_{\text{het}}}\right). \tag{7.8}$$

Basically this statistic compares the test statistic χ^2_{het} with its expectation under the homogeneity model. I^2 takes values between 0 and 1. The I^2 statistic may be interpreted as the variation in effect size attributable to heterogeneity For the data at hand I^2 is 0.6985, indicating strong heterogeneity. Recently Huedo-Medina et al. (2006) investigated the power of both procedures. Their results show the utility of the I^2 index as a complement to the χ^2_{het} test, although it has the same problems of power with a small number of studies. Recently, Jackson (2006) confirmed this well-known fact analytically from simulation studies (Jones et al. 1989).

A more powerful method is given by model-based approaches. A model-based approach has the advantage that it can be used to test specific alternatives and thus has higher power to detect heterogeneity. So far we have considered the following simple fixed effects model:

$$\hat{\theta}_i = \theta + \varepsilon_i, \quad i = 1, \ldots, k, \quad \varepsilon_i \sim N(0, \sigma_i^2). \tag{7.9}$$

Obviously, this model is not able to account for any heterogeneity, since deviations from $\hat{\theta}_i$ and θ are assumed to be explained only by random error.

Thus, alternatively, a random effects model which incorporates variation between studies should be considered. It is assumed that each study has its own (true) exposure effect and that there is a random distribution of these true exposure effects around a central effect. This idea is presented in Fig. 7.7. Frequently, it is assumed that the individual study effects follow a normal distribution with mean θ_i and variance σ_i^2 and the random distribution of the true effects is again a normal distribution with variance τ^2. In other words, the random effects model allows nonhomogeneity between the effects of different studies. This leads to the following model:

$$\hat{\theta}_i = \theta_i + \varepsilon_i = \theta + b_i + \varepsilon_i, \quad i = 1, \ldots, k, \tag{7.10}$$

with $\hat{\theta}_i \sim N(\theta, \tau^2 + \sigma_i^2), b_i \sim N(0, \tau^2), \varepsilon_i \sim N(0, \sigma_i^2)$. The observed effects from different studies are used to estimate the parameters describing the fixed and random effects. This may be done using maximum likelihood procedures (Brockwell and Gordon 2001; Hardy and Thompson 1996), methods of moments (DerSimonian

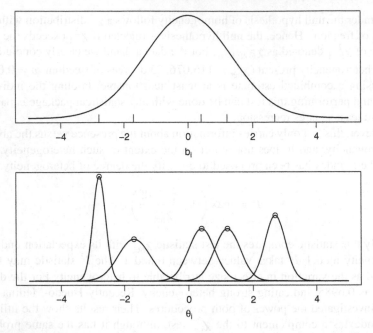

Fig. 7.7 Random effects model: variable effects drawn from a population of study effects

and Laird 1986), or an approach based on weighted least squares linear regression. In the following sections these approaches are described. Of particular importance is the estimation of the variability between studies which is quantified by the heterogeneity variance τ^2. To compare the performance of these methods, a simulation study was performed.

7.3.1 The DerSimonian–Laird Approach

The widely used approach by DerSimonian and Laird (1986) applies a method of moments to obtain an estimate of τ^2. Taking the expectation of (7.10) leads to

$$E(\hat{\theta}_i) = \theta$$

and calculating the variance leads to

$$\text{var}(\hat{\theta}_i) = \text{var}(b_i) + \text{var}(\varepsilon_i) = \tau^2 + \sigma_i^2 = \sigma_i^{*2},$$

assuming that b_i and ε_i are independent. The heterogeneity variance τ^2 is unknown and has to be estimated from the data. The method of DerSimonian and Laird equates the heterogeneity test statistic (7.7) to its expected value. This expectation is calculated under the assumption of a random effects model and is given by

$$E(\chi_{\text{het}}^2) = k - 1 + \tau^2 \left(\sum w_i - \frac{\sum w_i^2}{\sum w_i} \right).$$

The weights w_i are given by the inverse variance. Equating χ_{het}^2 to its expectation in the heterogeneity model and solving for τ^2 gives

$$\hat{\tau}^2 = \frac{\chi_{\text{het}}^2 - (k-1)}{\sum w_i - \frac{\sum w_i^2}{\sum w_i}}. \tag{7.11}$$

In the case $\chi_{\text{het}}^2 < k - 1$, the estimator $\hat{\tau}^2$ is truncated to zero. An advantage of the estimator (7.11) of τ is that a closed form is available and no iterative procedures are required. The estimator (7.11) of τ^2 will be denoted as the "DL estimator."

Under model (7.10) the variance of the study-specific effects θ_i is given by

$$\text{var}(\hat{\theta}_i) = \sigma_i^2 + \tau^2. \tag{7.12}$$

This follows directly from the result $\text{var}(Y) = E\left[\text{var}(Y|\lambda)\right] + \text{var}\left[E(Y|\lambda)\right]$ on the variance decomposition in (5.17) on page 120. Thus, instead of using weights $w_i = \frac{1}{\sigma_i^2}$, we need new weights with $w_i^* = \frac{1}{\sigma_i^2 + \tau^2}$ to compute the summary estimate $\hat{\theta}$. As a result, the pooled estimator $\hat{\theta}_{\text{DL}}$ under heterogeneity can be obtained as a weighted average using $\hat{\tau}^2$ as a plug-in estimate for τ^2:

$$\hat{\theta}_{\text{DL}} = \frac{\sum_{i=1}^k w_i^* \hat{\theta}_i}{\sum_{i=1}^k w_i^*}. \tag{7.13}$$

With

$$w_i^{*2} = \frac{1}{\sigma_i^{*2}} = \frac{1}{\hat{\tau}^2 + \sigma_i^2} \tag{7.14}$$

we obtain

$$\hat{\theta}_{\text{DL}} = \frac{\sum_{i=1}^k \hat{\theta}_i / (\hat{\tau}^2 + \sigma_i^2)}{\sum_{i=1}^k 1 / (\hat{\tau}^2 + \sigma_i^2)}. \tag{7.15}$$

The variance of this estimator is given by

$$\text{var}(\hat{\theta}_{\text{DL}}) = \frac{1}{\sum_{i=1}^k \frac{1}{\sigma_i^{*2}}}, \tag{7.16}$$

$$= \frac{1}{\sum_{i=1}^k \frac{1}{\hat{\tau}^2 + \sigma_i^2}}. \tag{7.17}$$

The between-study variance τ^2 can also be interpreted as a measure of heterogeneity between studies. It should be noted that, in general, random effects methods yield larger variance and confidence intervals than fixed effects models because a between-study component τ^2 is added to the variance. If the heterogeneity between the studies is large, τ^2 will dominate the weights and all studies will be weighted more equally (in random effects models weight decreases for larger studies compared with the fixed effects model). For our example we obtain a pooled DerSimonian–Laird estimate of $\hat{\theta}_{DL} = 0.0337$ with heterogeneity variance $\hat{\tau}^2 = 0.0453$. The variance of the pooled estimator is given by $\text{var}(\hat{\theta}_{DL}) = 0.0024$. Transformed back to the original scale we obtain an OR of 1.034 with 95% confidence interval (0.939–1.139). On the basis of this analysis we would conclude that after adjusting for heterogeneity this meta-analysis does not provide evidence for an association between HRT and breast cancer in women.

One comment is in order. Within the DerSimonian–Laird approach the study-specific variances are assumed to be known constants. This is one of the reasons why this method can lead to a considerable bias when pooling estimates as demonstrated by Böhning et al. (2002).

Besides the moment-based method of DerSimonian and Laird, estimates of τ^2 can be obtained using likelihood-based methods. See the tutorials by Normand (1999) and van Houwelingen et al. (2002) for an introduction. Both tutorials refer mainly to the use of the software package SAS for the estimation of τ^2 without methodological details. These details are developed in the next section.

7.3.2 Maximum Likelihood Estimation of the Heterogeneity Variance τ^2

Again, a random effects model is assumed. The likelihood to be maximized is given by

$$L(\hat{\theta}_i; \theta, \tau^2) = (2\pi)^{-\frac{k}{2}} \prod_{i=1}^{k} \left(\frac{1}{\sigma_i^2 + \tau^2} \right)^{\frac{1}{2}} \exp\left(-\frac{1}{2} \sum_{i=1}^{k} \frac{(\hat{\theta}_i - \theta)^2}{\sigma_i^2 + \tau^2} \right). \quad (7.18)$$

Applying logs and computing derivatives with respect to θ and τ^2 and equating them to 0 leads to the equations

$$\sum_{i=1}^{k} \frac{\hat{\theta}_i}{\sigma_i^2 + \tau^2} = \theta \sum_{i=1}^{k} \frac{1}{\sigma_i^2 + \tau^2}, \quad (7.19)$$

$$\sum \frac{1}{\sigma_i^2 + \tau^2} = \sum \frac{(\hat{\theta}_i - \theta)^2}{(\sigma_i^2 + \tau^2)^2}. \quad (7.20)$$

The estimate of the summary effect of all studies is then given by

$$\hat{\theta} = \frac{\sum_{i=1}^{k} w_i^* \hat{\theta}_i}{\sum_{i=1}^{k} w_i^*}, \quad w_i^* = \frac{1}{\sigma_i^2 + \tau^2} \quad i = 1, \ldots, k. \tag{7.21}$$

As before, the summary estimate is a weighted sum of individual estimates of the respective studies. Usually, the heterogeneity variance τ^2 is not known and needs to be estimated from the data.

Equation (7.20) has no closed-form solution. After some algebra (7.20) can be transformed into the following equation:

$$\hat{\tau}^2 = \frac{\sum w_i^{*2}((\hat{\theta}_i - \hat{\theta})^2 - \sigma_i^2)}{\sum w_i^{*2}} \quad i = 1, \ldots, k. \tag{7.22}$$

Based on (7.21) and (7.22), Algorithm 7.3.1 can be used to estimate τ^2.

Set $\hat{\tau}^2 = 0$ as the initial value

Step 1: Compute $\hat{\theta} = \frac{\sum_{i=1}^{k} \hat{\theta}_i / (\hat{\tau}^2 + \sigma_i^2)}{\sum_{i=1}^{k} 1 / (\hat{\tau}^2 + \sigma_i^2)}$

Step 2: Compute $\hat{\tau}^2 = \frac{\sum w_i^{*2}((\hat{\theta}_i - \hat{\theta})^2 - \sigma_i^2)}{\sum w_i^{*2}}$ $i = 1, \ldots, k.$ and go to step 1

Algorithm 7.3.1: Algorithm to compute the maximum likelihood estimate of τ^2

This procedure is repeated until convergence is achieved, e.g., when there is no further improvement of the log likelihood. We will refer to this estimator as the "ML estimator." For the breast cancer data an estimate of $\hat{\tau}^2 = 0.086$ is obtained. Estimates based on likelihood methods offer the advantage that they provide the option to formally test which model is appropriate for the data by applying the likelihood ratio test or penalized criteria such as the Bayesian information criterion (BIC). The BIC is obtained by the formula BIC $= -2 \times \log$ likelihood $+ \log(k) \times q$, where q is the number of parameters in the model and k denotes the number of studies. A comparison of various models is shown in Table 7.2.

Table 7.2 Estimates of τ^2 and model comparison for the breast cancer data

Method	Residual heterogeneity	Estimates (SE) intercept	Heterogeneity $(\hat{\tau}^2)$	$\log L$	BIC
Fixed	None	0.056 (0.023)	–	−33.19	70.0
Mixed	Additive	0.027 (0.061)	0.086	−18.65	44.4
FM	Additive	0.033	0.079	−17.63	53.2
DL	Additive	0.034	0.045		
SH	Additive	0.045	0.199		

SE standard error, *BIC* Bayesian information criterion, *FM* finite mixture, *DL* DerSimonian and Laird, *SH* simple heterogeneity

7.3.3 Another Estimator of τ^2: The Simple Heterogeneity Variance Estimator

Recently, Sidik and Jonkman (2005) proposed a simple method for the estimation of the heterogeneity variance τ^2. As before, they consider a random effects model as in (7.10) with $b_i \sim N(0, \tau^2)$. For the purpose of their estimation method they reparameterize the variance of

$$\text{var}(\hat{\theta}_i) = \tau^2 + \sigma_i^2 = \tau^2 \frac{\sigma_i^2 + \tau^2}{\tau^2} = \tau^2(r_i + 1),$$

with $r_i = \sigma_i^2 / \tau^2$. Then the problem of estimating τ^2 is cast into the framework of simple linear regression:

$$E(\hat{\theta}) = X\theta,$$
$$\text{var}(\hat{\theta}_1) = \tau^2 V. \tag{7.23}$$

Here, X is a vector of 1s with dimension $k \times 1$ and V is diagonal matrix with elements $r_1 + 1, \ldots, r_k + 1$. In the framework of the usual weighted least squares an estimate of θ is obtained as

$$\hat{\theta}_V = \frac{\sum_{i=1}^{k} v_i^{-1} \hat{\theta}_i}{\sum_{i=1}^{k} v_i^{-1}}, \tag{7.24}$$

with $v_i = r_i + 1$. Note that this is equivalent to (7.15) and (7.21). The advantage of casting the problem into the usual weighted least squares approach is that an estimate for τ^2 can be obtained as the usual weighted residual sum of squares as follows:

$$\tau^2 = \frac{1}{k-1} \sum_{i=1}^{k} v_i^{-1} (\hat{\theta}_i - \hat{\theta}_V)^2. \tag{7.25}$$

Of course an estimate of τ is needed to compute the ratios r_i of the within-study variance σ_i^2 and the between-study variance τ^2. Here, Sidik and Jonkman propose using the empirical variance of the study-specific estimates $\hat{\theta}_i$:

$$\hat{\tau}_0^2 = \frac{1}{k} \sum_{i=1}^{k} (\hat{\theta}_i - \bar{\theta})^2. \tag{7.26}$$

Plugging this into (7.25) leads to

$$\hat{\tau}_{\text{SH}}^2 = \frac{1}{k-1} \sum_{i=1}^{k} \hat{v}^{-1} (\hat{\theta}_i - \theta_V)^2, \tag{7.27}$$

with $\hat{v}_i = \hat{r}_i + 1$ and $\hat{r}_i = \sigma_i^2 / \hat{\tau}_0^2$. Note that this estimator is strictly positive, in contrast to the DL estimator. This estimator will be referred to as the simple heterogeneity (SH) variance estimator. For the data at hand an estimate for $\hat{\tau}^2$ is 0.199.

7.3.4 A Comment on Summary Estimates Under Heterogeneity

Pooling in the presence of heterogeneity may be seriously misleading. As already outlined in Chap. 2, medicine tries to reach individualized therapy and as a result population-averaged estimates are not particularly helpful. Heterogeneity between studies should yield careful investigation of the sources of the differences. If there are a sufficient number of different studies available, further analyses, such as "metaregression," may be used to examine the sources of heterogeneity (Greenland 1987, 1994). Sometimes it seems more fruitful to consider a meta-analysis as a "study over studies" rather than to summarize a number of studies in a single number plus confidence interval. A natural approach for treating a meta-analysis as a study over studies is the finite mixture model approach since it allows classification of the individual study. This categorization may then be used to learn more specific aspects of the individual studies, leading to heterogeneity of effects.

7.3.5 The Finite Mixture Model Approach

When random effects models are used, another topic of interest is the form of the random effects' distribution. Besides a parametric distribution for the random effects, a discrete distribution may be assumed. Here we suppose that the study-specific estimators $\hat{\theta}_1, \hat{\theta}_2, \ldots, \hat{\theta}_k$ come from q subpopulations θ_j, $j = 1, \ldots, q$. Again, assuming that the effect of each individual study follows a normal distribution,

$$f(\hat{\theta}_i, \theta_j) = \frac{1}{\sqrt{2\pi\sigma_i^2}} \exp\left[-\frac{(\hat{\theta}_i - \theta_j)^2}{2\sigma_i^2}\right], \quad j = 1, \ldots, q, \qquad (7.28)$$

Note that (7.28) is the nonparametric discrete random effects analogue to (7.10), where a continuous parametric distribution is assumed for the random effects.

This leads to a finite mixture model with

$$f(\hat{\theta}_i, P) = \sum_{j=1}^{q} p_j f(\hat{\theta}_i, \theta_j, \sigma_i^2). \qquad (7.29)$$

The parameters of the mixing distribution P are

$$P = \begin{bmatrix} \theta_1 & \cdots & \theta_q \\ p_1 & \cdots & p_q. \end{bmatrix}, \quad \text{with} \quad p_j \geq 0 \quad j = 1, \ldots, q, \qquad (7.30)$$

$$p_1 + \cdots + p_q = 1. \qquad (7.31)$$

These parameters need to be estimated from the data. The mixing weights p_j denote the a priori probability of an observation belonging to a certain subpopulation with parameter θ_j. Note that the number of components q needs to be estimated as

Table 7.3 Finite mixture model for the breast cancer data

Components	Parameter $\hat{\theta}_j$	Weights $\hat{p}_j$	$\log L$
1	0.0056	1	−33.191
2	−0.3367	0.280	−22.863
	0.1137	0.720	
	−0.3365	0.2804	
3	0.0778	0.5671	−17.631
	0.5446	0.1524	

well. Estimation may be done with the program C.A.MAN (Böhning et al. 1998; Schlattmann and Bohning 1993). Alternatively, the software package META especially developed by the author (Schlattmann et al. 2003) for meta-analysis could be applied to estimate the parameters of the mixture model. Additionally the R package CAMAN can be used, which provides the functionality of C.A.MAN within an R library. For the HRT data we find a solution with the three components shown in Table 7.3 which provides a much better fit to the data than a fixed effects model.
  Here, the weights correspond to the mixing weights p_j and the parameter corresponds to the subpopulation mean θ_j, $j = 1,\ldots,q$. These results imply that about 28% of the studies show a protective effect of HRT, whereas the majority of the studies show a harmful effect. About 57% of the studies show an increased risk of 0.08 and 15% of the studies show a $\log$ (OR) of 0.54 Thus, using a finite mixture model, we find again considerable heterogeneity where the majority of studies find a harmful effect of HRT. It is noteworthy that some of the studies find a beneficial effect. Of course this needs to be investigated further. One way to do this is to classify the individual studies using the finite mixture model. Doing so, we find that for the example study nine of the data given in Table 7.1 belong to this category. This is a case-control study for which no information about confounder adjustment is available. This would be a starting point for a sensitivity analysis.

Estimation of the Heterogeneity Variance τ^2

On the basis of the finite mixture model, an estimate of the heterogeneity variance τ^2 is given by

$$\hat{\tau}^2 = \sum_{j=1}^{\hat{q}} \hat{p}_j \left(\hat{\theta}_j - \bar{\theta}\right)^2, \quad \text{with} \quad \bar{\theta} = \sum_{j=1}^{\hat{q}} \hat{p}_j\hat{\theta}_j. \tag{7.32}$$

Note that the special case of $\hat{q} = 1$ denotes the fixed effects model with a corresponding heterogeneity variance $\tau^2 = 0$. For our example an estimate of 0.079 is obtained using this approach.

Table 7.2 gives an overview of the models fitted so far. These include the fixed effects model with a BIC of 70.0 and the mixed effects model using a normal distribution for the random effects with a BIC of 44.4. The finite mixture model has a BIC value of 53.2. Thus, from the data in Table 7.2 it is quite obvious that a fixed effects model does not fit the data well and that a random effects model should be used. Of course, the question remains which random effects model should be chosen for the analysis. Solely based on the likelihood, the finite mixture model provides a slightly better fit than the linear mixed effects model. However, based on the BIC given in Table 7.2, one would choose the parametric mixture model provided the assumption of a normal distribution of the random effects is justifiable. This can be investigated, for example, by a normal quantile–quantile plot of the estimated individual random effects given by the parametric model. This will be presented later when using metaregression methods.

In terms of the estimates of the heterogeneity variance τ^2 a large variability is observable. The smallest estimate of τ^2 is given by the method of DerSimonian and Laird, with a value of 0.045 for $\hat{\tau}^2$. Then follows the finite mixture model estimate, with a value of $\tau^2 = 0.079$, and then the linear mixed model, with an estimate of $\hat{\tau}^2 = 0.086$. The largest estimate is given by the SH variance, with $\hat{\tau}^2 = 0.199$. Clearly, this variability raises the question of which estimator should be applied in practical data analysis.

7.4 A Simulation Study Comparing Four Estimators of τ^2

To assess the performance of the various estimators a simulation study was performed. This study compared the finite mixture model approach, the SH variance estimator, the ML estimator based on the normal distribution for the random effects, and the DL estimator. The simulation study investigated bias, standard deviation, and mean square error (MSE) for all four estimators of τ^2.

7.4.1 Design of the Simulation Study

To provide comparability with simulation studies from the literature, the simulation set-up of Sidik and Jonkman (2005) was applied in this study. Five meta-analysis sample sizes were chosen, with $k = 10$, 20, 30, 50, and 80. The true overall effect of θ was set to be 0.5. Eight values of τ^2 were considered, specifically $\tau^2 = 0.10$, 0.25, 0.50, 0.75, 1.00, 1.25, 1.50, and 2.00. For each combination of k and τ^2 and θ 2×2 tables were generated for given k. This method was proposed by Berkey et al. (1995) and was also applied by Platt et al. (1999) and Knapp and Hartung (2003). In the first step θ_i was generated from $N(0, \tau^2)$ for $i = 1, \ldots, k$. For a given k the sample n_{iC} of the control groups were randomly chosen from the integers 20, 21,

22,...,200. In addition, the sample sizes for the treatment groups were randomly chosen from the integers $30, 31, \ldots, 300$. The responses for the control group were generated from a binomial distribution $\mathrm{Bin}(n_{iC}, p_{iC})$, where the binomial probability p_{iC} was randomly chosen from a uniform distribution on the interval 0.05–0.65. The responses x_{iT} for the treatment were generated from a binomial distribution $\mathrm{Bin}(n_{iT}, p_{iT})$ with

$$p_{iT} = p_{iC} \exp(\theta_i)/(1 - p_{iC} + p_{iC} \exp(\theta_i)) \quad i = 1, \ldots, k.$$

With use of this method k 2×2 tables were generated. From cell counts of the ith table denoted by $a_i = x_{iT}$, $b_i = n_{iC} - x_{iC}$, $c_i = n_{iT} - x_{iT}$, $d_i = x_{iC}$ log (ORs) for the ith study with corresponding variance estimates were calculated as

$$\hat{\theta}_i = \log \frac{(a_i + 0.5)(d_i + 0.5)}{(c_i + 0.5)(d_i + 0.5)},$$

$$\hat{\sigma}_i^2 = \frac{1}{a_i + 0.5} + \frac{1}{b_i + 0.5} + \frac{1}{c_i + 0.5} + \frac{1}{d_i + 0.5}.$$

As before, the estimates σ^2 are treated as constants and not as random variables. For these simulated data an estimate of the heterogeneity variance τ^2 was obtained using the method of DerSimonian and Laird (7.11) , the maximum likelihood estimate (Algorithm 7.3.1), the finite mixture model (7.32), and the SH variance (7.27). Using finite mixture models the number of components q needs to be estimated as well. For the purpose of this simulation study the mixture algorithm (Algorithm 4.4.2) on page 79 was used. This algorithm gives an estimate of the number of components by combining the vertex exchange method (VEM) algorithm (Algorithm 4.3.2) and the expectation maxmization (EM) algorithm (Algorithm 4.4.1). An advantage of this algorithm lies in the fact that the number of components q must not be specified in advance. The VEM algorithm identifies population means θ_j with positive support which may coincide using the EM algorithm. Thus, this algorithm provides an estimate of the number of components q, the mixing weights p_j, and population means θ_j which are then used to estimate τ^2.

The whole procedure was replicated $N = 20,000$ times. From the N estimates, the mean, the standard deviation, the bias, and the MSE for each of the four methods are calculated as

$$\mathrm{Bias} = \frac{1}{N} \sum_{i=1}^{N} \hat{\tau}_i^2 - \tau^2, \tag{7.33}$$

$$\mathrm{Variance} = \frac{1}{N} \sum_{i=1}^{N} (\hat{\tau}_i^2 - \bar{\tau}^2)^2, \tag{7.34}$$

$$\mathrm{MSE} = \frac{1}{N} \sum_{i=1}^{N} (\hat{\tau}_i^2 - \tau^2)^2. \tag{7.35}$$

Software and Computing Facilities

The algorithms and the simulation studies were programmed in C++ using the GNU GCC 3.3.5-5 compiler. Random numbers were generated using portable random number generators using C code provided by L'Ecuyer (1988). The programs made use of a PC UNIX(Linux) system. Plots were produced using the statistical computing package R (R Development Core Team 2008), which is a freely available clone of the commercial package S-plus.

7.4.2 Simulation Results

The results of the simulation study performed to investigate the accuracy of the four heterogeneity variance estimators are shown in Table 7.4. The most notable results of the simulation study are given in terms of bias. From Table 7.4 it can be seen that the SH estimator offers the best performance with respect to bias. Especially for large heterogeneity variances τ^2 the SH variance has the smallest bias, whereas the other estimators underestimate τ^2. The second-best estimator in terms of bias is based on the finite mixture model, which provides a smaller bias in comparison with the linear mixed effect model estimates and the DL estimator. With increasing heterogeneity variance τ^2, the bias of the DL estimator increases dramatically in magnitude, especially for values of τ^2 greater than or equal to 0.75. This applies to all meta-analysis sample sizes with the exception of $k = 10$ and $k = 20$. As may be seen also from Fig. 7.8 the linear mixed effects model estimator has smaller bias than the DL estimator but larger bias than the finite mixture model and the SH variance estimator. For increasing k and τ^2 the bias of the ML estimator increases.

Evaluating the estimators in terms of the MSE, it is apparent that the values depend on τ^2 and the number of studies k. For a large value of τ^2, i.e., $\tau^2 \geq 0.75$, and $k \geq 50$ the SH estimator has a smaller MSE than the other estimators. In this setting the MSEs of the finite mixture model and the linear mixed effects model provide reasonable estimates, whereas the MSE of the DL estimator increases greatly. For large values of k and small values of τ, all estimators have similar MSEs.

Overall, the SH variance estimator has acceptable bias and MSE. The second-best estimator in terms of bias and variance is given by the finite mixture model, followed by the linear mixed effects model. The DL estimator has unfavorable bias and MSEs for larger values of k and τ.

7.4.3 Discussion

On the basis of this simulation one would recommend the SH estimator as the method of choice to compute the heterogeneity variance τ^2 in a meta-analysis. This is in line with the results of the simulation study performed by Sidik and Jonkman

Table 7.4 Empirical statistics of four estimators of τ^2 based on N simulation replicates

k	τ^2	Bias				MSE			
		FM	ML	SH	DL	FM	ML	SH	DL
10	0.10	0.004	−0.022	0.037	−0.003	0.008	0.006	0.009	0.007
	0.25	−0.013	−0.049	0.021	−0.018	0.025	0.023	0.026	0.025
	0.50	−0.037	−0.086	0.007	−0.049	0.074	0.070	0.079	0.072
	0.75	−0.068	−0.129	−0.008	−0.099	0.144	0.139	0.158	0.135
	1.00	−0.105	−0.176	−0.027	−0.164	0.241	0.233	0.265	0.219
	1.25	−0.135	−0.220	−0.037	−0.233	0.361	0.350	0.398	0.324
	1.50	−0.173	−0.273	−0.056	−0.321	0.511	0.490	0.558	0.450
	2.00	−0.251	−0.374	−0.090	−0.513	0.856	0.837	0.944	0.785
20	0.10	0.001	−0.016	0.037	−0.006	0.004	0.004	0.005	0.004
	0.25	−0.009	−0.032	0.021	−0.019	0.012	0.012	0.013	0.012
	0.50	−0.028	−0.059	0.006	−0.054	0.037	0.036	0.037	0.035
	0.75	−0.051	−0.090	−0.008	−0.106	0.072	0.072	0.074	0.069
	1.00	−0.075	−0.122	−0.022	−0.172	0.122	0.121	0.126	0.117
	1.25	−0.102	−0.160	−0.036	−0.254	0.183	0.182	0.188	0.184
	1.50	−0.135	−0.202	−0.054	−0.345	0.256	0.255	0.262	0.273
	2.00	−0.208	−0.292	−0.097	−0.556	0.424	0.434	0.433	0.534
30	0.10	−0.000	−0.013	0.037	−0.007	0.003	0.002	0.004	0.002
	0.25	−0.009	−0.025	0.022	−0.018	0.008	0.008	0.008	0.008
	0.50	−0.029	−0.052	0.003	−0.057	0.024	0.024	0.024	0.024
	0.75	−0.049	−0.079	−0.010	−0.111	0.050	0.050	0.049	0.050
	1.00	−0.071	−0.107	−0.022	−0.178	0.081	0.083	0.082	0.088
	1.25	−0.101	−0.143	−0.040	−0.261	0.122	0.125	0.122	0.145
	1.50	−0.130	−0.178	−0.057	−0.352	0.173	0.177	0.172	0.224
	2.00	−0.208	−0.270	−0.104	−0.574	0.297	0.311	0.292	0.474
50	0.10	−0.002	−0.011	0.036	−0.007	0.001	0.001	0.003	0.001
	0.25	−0.009	−0.020	0.023	−0.018	0.005	0.005	0.005	0.005
	0.50	−0.026	−0.042	0.007	−0.056	0.015	0.015	0.015	0.016
	0.75	−0.048	−0.068	−0.010	−0.112	0.031	0.032	0.029	0.035
	1.00	−0.069	−0.094	−0.022	−0.181	0.050	0.052	0.049	0.066
	1.25	−0.098	−0.126	−0.040	−0.264	0.077	0.080	0.073	0.115
	1.50	−0.129	−0.161	−0.058	−0.359	0.110	0.116	0.105	0.188
	2.00	−0.208	−0.247	−0.107	−0.583	0.193	0.206	0.177	0.424
80	0.10	−0.004	−0.009	0.036	−0.007	0.001	0.001	0.002	0.001
	0.25	−0.011	−0.019	0.022	−0.019	0.003	0.003	0.003	0.003
	0.50	−0.028	−0.039	0.005	−0.058	0.009	0.010	0.009	0.011
	0.75	−0.049	−0.063	−0.010	−0.113	0.020	0.021	0.018	0.027
	1.00	−0.072	−0.089	−0.025	−0.184	0.033	0.035	0.030	0.054
	1.25	−0.102	−0.121	−0.044	−0.270	0.052	0.055	0.046	0.101
	1.50	−0.132	−0.153	−0.060	−0.364	0.074	0.079	0.065	0.168
	2.00	−0.213	−0.237	−0.111	−0.590	0.138	0.147	0.114	0.400

MSE mean square error, *FM* finite mixture model, *ML* maximum likelihood estimator, *SH* simple heterogeneity variance, *DL* DerSimonian–Laird estimator

(2005), who also found the SH variance estimator is superior to the DL estimator. Since this method is easily extended to include covariates, as it is a special case of weighted linear regression, it could easily be used for metaregression.

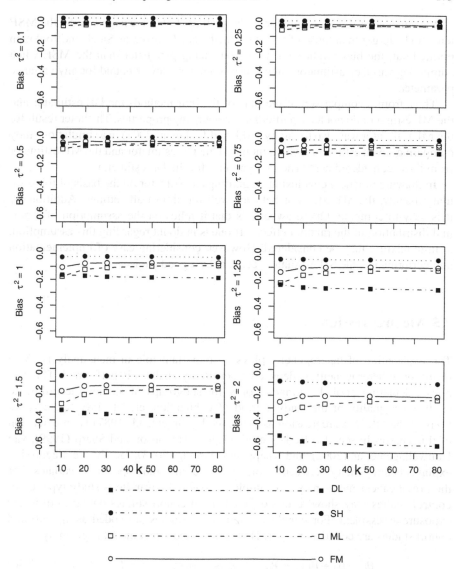

Fig. 7.8 Bias of four estimates of the heterogeneity variance τ^2. *FM* a finite mixture model, *ML* the maximum likelihood estimator, *SH* the simple heterogeneity variance, *DL* the DerSimonian–Laird estimator

Another method to compute the heterogeneity variance is based on finite mixture models. This method performs second best in terms of bias and MSE, but tends to underestimate τ^2 for large τ and k. On the other hand, no distributional assumption about the form of the random effects distribution has to be made. Unfortunately the estimation of the model parameters cannot be obtained using a simple closed formula as for the SH estimator.

For small sizes the DL estimator has a small MSE, but for large k and τ the MSE tends to be larger than those of the other methods. However, as Sidek and Jonkman pointed out, the bias might be a more convincing parameter than the MSE when comparing variance estimators since zero is a natural lower bound for any variance parameter.

Thus, from a comparison of the bias of the four methods the DL estimator and the ML estimator do not have particularly convincing properties. The latter result for the ML estimator was also found by Sidik and Jonkman (2007) in a simulation study comparing seven estimators which included the DL estimator and the ML estimator from those considered here. The same applies for the DL estimator.

In drawing practical conclusions regarding an estimator on the basis of this simulation study, the SH estimator behaves well for almost all settings. Additionally it is easy to compute. One drawback is that it relies on the assumption of a normal distribution of the random effects. If one is in doubt regarding this assumption, a finite mixture may be considered. However, considering ease of implementation and performance, the SH estimator seems to be a good choice.

7.5 Metaregression

The explanation of heterogeneity plays an important role in meta-analysis. As a result, once heterogeneity is detected a sensitivity analysis is performed. This implies calculating pooled estimators only for subgroups of studies (according to study type, quality of the study, period of publication, etc.) to investigate variations of the OR. Metaregression as proposed by Greenland (1987) is an extension of this approach; see also Berkey et al. (1995), Thompson and Sharp (1999), van Houwelingen et al. (2002), and Knapp and Hartung (2003). Ideally, metaregression explains heterogeneity between studies by including study-specific covariates. For the breast cancer meta-analysis example, a potential covariate is study type; case-control studies may show results different from cohort studies owing to different exposure assessment. For our data case-control studies are coded as $x_{i1} = 0$ and cohort studies are coded as $x_{i1} = 1$. Hence, the fixed effect model is given by

$$\hat{\theta}_i = \beta_0 + \beta_1 x_{i1} + \varepsilon_i, \qquad \varepsilon_i \sim N(0, \sigma_i^2), \quad i = 1, \ldots, k. \qquad (7.36)$$

Here, based on the regression equation $\hat{\theta}_i = 0.0015 + 0.145 x_i$, we find that cohort studies show an association between HRT and breast cancer. Obviously, cohort studies provide results different from case-control studies. Clearly, after adjustment for covariates the question remains of whether there is still residual heterogeneity present. Again, we can analyze the data using a random effects model in this case with a random intercept:

$$\hat{\theta}_i = \beta_0 + \beta_1 x_{i1} + b_i + \varepsilon_i, \qquad b_i \sim N(0, \tau^2), \quad \varepsilon_i \sim N(0, \sigma_i^2). \qquad (7.37)$$

For this model the regression equation for the fixed effects is $\hat{\theta}_i = -0.009 + 0.1080x_{i1}$ for a cohort study and the corresponding heterogeneity variance is estimated as $\hat{\tau}^2 = 0.079$ by the maximum likelihood method.

On the basis of model (7.37), the estimates of the random effects b_i are obtained by

$$E(b_i|\hat{\theta}_i) = \frac{\tau^2}{\sigma_i^2 + \tau^2}(\hat{\theta}_i - (\beta_0 + \beta_1 x_{i1})).$$

Immediately, there is the serious problem that τ^2, β_0, and β_1 are not known. Plugging their estimates into (7.38) leads to the following empirical Bayes estimates of b_i:

$$\hat{b}_i = \frac{\hat{\tau}^2}{\sigma_i^2 + \hat{\tau}^2}(\hat{\theta}_i - (\hat{\beta}_0 + \hat{\beta}_1 x_i)). \tag{7.38}$$

From the factor $\hat{\tau}^2/(\sigma_i^2 + \hat{\tau}^2)$ it is clear that $\hat{b}_i$ is a weighted average of zero (the prior mean of b_i) and the residual $r_i = \hat{\theta} - \hat{\beta}_0 - \hat{\beta}_1 x_i$. Equation (7.38) also shows that shrinkage will be large for studies with a large study-specific variance.

Besides the ML estimators (Hardy and Thompson 1996) used here, several estimators for τ^2 are available. See, for example, a confidence interval based approach proposed by Knapp et al. (2006).

7.5.1 Finite Mixture Models Adjusted for Covariates

Again, instead of a parametric distribution for the random effects a discrete distribution can be assumed. Instead of a parametric mixture, a finite mixture model adjusted for covariates can be applied. We have the same semiparametric mixing distribution as in (3.13) on page 33:

$$P = \begin{bmatrix} \lambda_1 & \cdots & \lambda_q \\ p_1 & \cdots & p_q \end{bmatrix}. \tag{7.39}$$

The major difference is now that parameters $\lambda_1, \ldots, \lambda_q$ are no longer scalar quantities but are vectors, e.g.,

$$\lambda_1 = (\beta_{01}, \beta_{11}, \ldots, \beta_{m1}), \tag{7.40}$$

where m denotes the number of covariates in the model. In contrast to the homogenous case we have the same type of density f for each subpopulation but a different parameter vector λ_j in subpopulation j. The expectation of the ith observation in the jth subpopulation is then given by

$$E(\theta_{ij}) = x_i\lambda_j = \beta_{0j} + \beta_{1j}x_{i1} + \cdots + \beta_{mj}x_{im}. \tag{7.41}$$

Table 7.5 Covariate-adjusted finite mixture model for the breast cancer data

Component	Weight p_j	Estimate	Standard error	t
Intercept 1	0.239	−0.386	0.066	−5.867
Intercept 2	0.614	0.035	0.029	1.211
Intercept 3	0.147	0.484	0.086	5.601
Type		0.097	0.044	2.201

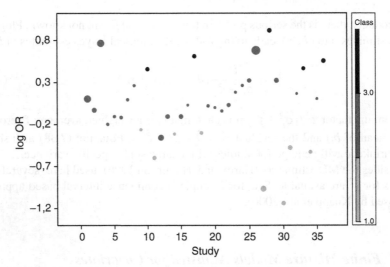

Fig. 7.9 Bubble plot of the breast cancer data with the individual studies categorized on the basis of a covariate-adjusted mixture model

In the simplest case a discrete random distribution only for the intercepts is assumed:

$$\theta_{ij} = \beta_j + \beta_1 x_{i1} + \varepsilon_i, \quad \varepsilon_i \sim N(0, \sigma_i^2). \tag{7.42}$$

The results found by the EM algorithm (Algorithm 4.6.4) for the covariate-adjusted mixture model are given in Table 7.5.

As before some of the studies seem to identify a beneficial effect of HRT, while a large proportion of the studies reveal only a small effect of 0.035 on the log scale with a corresponding OR of 1.036. About 15% of the studies find an OR of 1.642. Thus, after the inclusion of the covariate study type only little heterogeneity could be explained.

The probabilities e_{ij} which indicate the probability of the ith study belonging to jth component which are obtained in the estimation process of the mixture model (see (4.73) on page 92) can be used to classify the individual study using a maximum rule, i.e., the ith study is classified into that category for which the posterior probability e_{ij} is the highest. This idea is applied to the breast cancer data and is shown in Fig. 7.9.

Table 7.6 Comparison of fixed and random effects models

Method	Residual hetero.	Estimates (SE) intercept	Slope	Heterogeneity ($\hat{\tau}^2$)	BIC
Fixed effects model 1	None	0.056 (0.023)	–	–	70.0
Linear mixed effects 1	Additive	0.027 (0.061)	–	0.086	44.4
Fixed effects model 2	None	0.001 (0.029)	0.145 (0.046)	–	63.9
Linear mixed effects 2	Additive	−0.009 (0.072)	0.108 (0.126)	0.081	47.3
Finite mixture model 1	Additive	0.033 (–)	–	0.079	53.2
Finite mixture model 2	Additive	0.003 (–)	0.097 (0.044)	0.071	53.7

Table 7.6 compares fixed and random effects models for the HRT data. The table shows models with and without an estimate for the slope. Model selection can be based again on the BIC. Apparently, on the basis of BIC both fixed effects models do not fit the data very well since their BIC values are considerably higher than those of the random effects models. Note that if only the fixed effects models were considered this meta-analysis would show a harmful effect. In the fixed effects metaregression model this would apply only to cohort studies.

Comparing both linear mixed effects models which are based on the assumption of a normal distribution of the random effects the model with the covariate does not provide an improved fit of the data. The log likelihood is only slightly larger and penalizing the number of parameters leads to a larger BIC for the mixed effects model with the covariate.

Another interesting point is to compare the heterogeneity variance estimated by both models. Here, no substantial portion of heterogeneity is explained by the covariate, since the heterogeneity variance is reduced to 0.081 from 0.086. The same applies for the models where a discrete distribution is assumed for the random effects. Owing to the larger number of parameters which have to be estimated here the BIC values are larger. Thus, if the assumption of a normal distribution for the random effects is satisfied, judging from the BIC we would choose the model with random intercept based on a normal distribution for the random effects. To investigate the normality of the random effects Fig. 7.10 shows a quantile–quantile plot of the estimated random effects. According to Fig. 7.10 the assumption of a normal distribution seems to be compatible with the data, although there is a slight indication of departure from normality at the tails. As a result, the normal random effects model (intercepts only) would be chosen.

These conclusions are merely data-driven; thus, from a statistical point of view further covariates need to be identified and included in the model. From a public health point of view the conclusion is perhaps less straightforward. Although inclusion of the covariate study type does not explain the heterogeneity of the studies very well, we find that cohort studies find a harmful effect. One might argue that although these results are far from perfect they should not be ignored as absence of evidence does not imply evidence of absence. Looking back at these data in the light of the results from the Women's Health Initiative study (Rossouw et al. 2002),

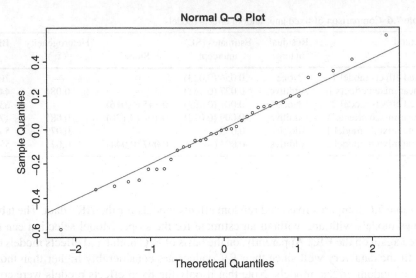

Fig. 7.10 Normal quantile–quantile plot for estimated random effects

it becomes clear that caution is required in the analysis and interpretation of meta-analyses of observational studies. The major finding of the Women's Health Initiative study was that the group of subjects undergoing treatment with combined HRT in the form of PREMPRO (0.625 mg/day conjugated equine estrogens + 2.5 mg/day medroxyprogesterone acetate) was found to have an increased risk of breast cancer (hazard ratio 1.26, 95% confidence interval 1.00–1.59) and no apparent cardiac benefit. This is contradictory to the prior belief that HRT provides cardiovascular benefit. As a result, although several benefits were considered, these interim findings at 5 years were deemed sufficiently troubling to stop this arm of the trial after 5.2 years.

7.6 Interpretation of the Results of Meta-analysis of Observational Studies

The example in the previous section shows that the interpretation of the results of a meta-analysis should not only discuss the pooled estimator and the confidence interval but should also focus on the examination of the heterogeneity between the results of the studies. Strengths and weaknesses as well as potential bias should be discussed.

7.6.1 Bias

For epidemiologic studies in general, the main problem is not the lack of preci- sion and the random error but the fact that the results may be distorted by different sources of bias or confounding; for a general overview of the problem of bias, see Hill and Kleinbaum (2000). That means that the standard error (or the size of the study) may not be the best indicator for the weight of a study. If more or better data are collected on a smaller number of subjects, the results may be more accurate than in a large study with insufficient information on the risk factors or on confounders. The assessment of bias in individual studies is therefore crucial for the overall inter- pretation.

The central problem of meta-analyses of clinical trials is publication bias. It was the topic of a paper by Berlin et al. (1989) as early as 1989 and is still a topic of recent methodological investigations; see, for example, Copas and Shi (2001). This bias has received a lot of attention particularly in the area of clinical trials. Publica- tion bias occurs if studies that have nonsignificant or negative results are published less frequently than studies that have positive results. For randomized clinical trials, it has been shown that even with a computer-aided literature search only some of the relevant studies will be identified (Dickersin et al. 1994). For epidemiologic obser- vational studies additional problems exist, because often a large number of variables will be collected in questionnaires as potential confounders (Blettner et al. 1999). If one or several of these potential confounders yield significant or important results, they may be published in additional papers, which have often not been planned in advance. In general, publication bias yields a nonnegligible overestimation of the risk estimate.

However, as has been pointed out, there exist few systematic investigations of the magnitude of the problem for epidemiologic studies. A major worry is that non- significant results are neither mentioned in the title nor in the abstract and publica- tions may be lost in the retrieval process.

7.6.2 Confounding

Another problem arises because different studies adjust for different confounding factors. It is well known that the estimated effect of a factor of interest is (strongly) influenced by the inclusion or exclusion of other factors if these factors have an influence on the outcome and if they are correlated with the risk factor of interest. Combining estimates from several studies with different ways of adjusting for con- founders yields biased results. If only literature data are used, crude estimates may be available for some of the studies and model-based estimates for others. However, as the adjustment for confounders is an important issue for the assessment of an effect in each single study, it is obvious that combining these different estimates in a meta-analysis may not give meaningful results. It is necessary to use "similar" con- founders in each study to adjust the estimated effect of interest in the single studies.

In general that would require a reanalysis of the individual study. Obviously, that requires the original data and a meta-analysis with individual patient data is needed for this purpose.

7.6.3 Heterogeneity

In epidemiologic research different study designs are in use and none of them can be considered as a gold standard compared with the randomized clinical trial for therapy studies. Therefore, it is necessary to evaluate the comparability of the individual designs before summarizing the results. Often, case-control studies, cohort studies, and cross-sectional studies are used to investigate the same questions and results of those studies need to be combined. Egger et al. (2001) pointed out several examples in which results from case-control studies differ from those of cohort studies. For example, in a paper by Boyd et al. (1993), it was noted that cohort studies show no association between breast cancer and saturated fat intake, while the same meta-analysis using results from case-control studies only revealed an increased, statistically significant risk. Other reasons for heterogeneity may be different uses of data collection methods, different control selection (e.g., hospital vs. population controls), and differences in case ascertainment. Differences could be explored in a formal sensitivity analysis, but also by graphical methods (forest plot). However, meta-analyses from published data provide only limited information if the reasons for heterogeneity are to be investigated in depth. The problem of heterogeneity can be well demonstrated with nearly any example of a published meta-analysis. For example, Ursin et al. (1995) investigated the influence of the body mass index (BMI) on the development of premenopausal breast cancer. They included 23 studies, of which 19 were case-control studies and four were cohort studies. Some of these studies were designed to investigate BMI as a risk factor; others measured BMI as confounders in studies investigating other risk factors. One can speculate that the number of unpublished studies in which BMI was mainly considered as a confounder and did not show a strong influence on premenopausal breast cancer is nonnegligible and that this issue may result in some bias. As is usual practice in epidemiologic studies, relative risks were provided for several categories of BMI. To overcome this problem the authors estimated a regression coefficient for the relative risk as a function of the BMI; however, several critical assumptions are necessary for this type of approach. The authors found severe heterogeneity across all studies combined (the p value of a corresponding test was almost zero). An influence of the type of study (cohort study or case-control study) was apparent; therefore, no overall summary was presented for case-control and cohort studies combined. One reason for the heterogeneity may be the variation in adjustment for confounders. Adjustment for confounders other than age was used only in ten of the 23 studies.

7.7 Case Study: Aspirin Use and Breast Cancer Risk – A Meta-analysis and Metaregression of Observational Studies from 2001 to 2007

7.7.1 Introduction

With a prevalence of about 4.4 million women and a lethality rate of more than 410,000 cases per year, breast cancer is the most common cancer and the leading cause of death in women worldwide (Parkin et al. 2005; WHO 2002).

This large public health burden calls for preventive measures. One such potential preventive action might be chemoprevention given by regular intake of Aspirin or similar drugs.

Cyclooxygenase (COX) is an enzyme that is responsible for formation of biological mediators called prostanoids, which include prostaglandins, prostacyclin, and thromboxane. COX has two isonenzmyes: COX-1 and COX-2. COX-1 is considered a constitutive enzyme found in most mammalian cells. On the other hand, COX-2 is considered an inducible enzyme becoming abundant in inflammation. Pharmacological inhibition of COX-2 leads to symptom relief of inflammation and pain. This is the method of action of well-known drugs such as Aspirin and Ibuprofen, known as nonsteroidal anti-inflammatory drugs (NSAIDs). In the last few years, there has been an increasing body of evidence supporting the role of COX-2 in breast cancer development and progression (Arun and Goss 2004; Denkert et al. 2004; Vainio 1998). Aspirin and other NSAIDs are well-known inhibitors of COX and are therefore attractive agents for a potential chemoprevention in breast cancer. Animal and in vitro studies showed that NSAIDs are able to inhibit breast cancer cells and to suppress tumor growth (Harris et al. 2000; McCormick et al. 1985). Consequently, several observational studies were carried out but they provided inconsistent results. Two meta-analyses have been conducted that calculated a pooled risk reduction of 18% (Khuder and Mutgi 2001) and 23% (Gonzalez-Perez et al. 2003), respectively, for NSAID intake (relative risk 0.82, 95% confidence interval 0.66–0.88) and a relative risk of 0.77 (95% confidence interval 0.69–0.86) for Aspirin alone (Khuder and Mutgi 2001). It remains unclear which exposure categories were used to calculate the pooled relative risk and which criteria were used to chose them. Moreover, the reasons for heterogeneity between the individual studies and the dose-response relationship between NSAID intake and breast cancer risk were not examined. A review by Harris et al. (2005) dealt with dose response but took only frequency and not duration of use into account. Mangiapane, Blettner, and Schlattmann (2008) examined recent epidemiologic studies on Aspirin use and breast cancer published from 2001 to 2005, to investigate reasons for heterogeneity between the individual studies and to analyze a dose-response relationship considering frequency and duration of use. The analysis presented here is an extension of this meta-analysis incorporating studies until December 2007.

7.7.2 Literature Search and Data Extraction

We searched for published and unpublished literature evaluating the association between Aspirin and breast cancer risk. We systematically searched for cohort studies and case-control studies in the MEDLINE, CANCERLIT, and EMBASE databases for the period from January 1, 2001 to December 31, 2007. The search was restricted to publications in English and German. Medical subject headings (MeSH) and keywords used for the MEDLINE search were "Aspirin" or "anti-inflammatory drugs" or "NSAIDs" for the exposure and "breast cancer" for the outcome. The same keywords were used for the CANCERLIT and EMBASE search. Studies were included if they met the following criteria: (1) cohort study or case-control study; (2) evaluated the association between Aspirin and breast cancer; (3) reported a relative risk or odds ratio (OR) including confidence intervals or information to permit their calculation. Studies which investigated different types of NSAIDs were excluded if they did not present stratified estimates for Aspirin use alone. We checked references cited in original or review articles that were not found by the database search. To find unpublished material we contacted the authors of the epidemiologic literature in this field if their e-mail addresses were available. Additionally, we checked the Web sites of the American Society of Clinical Oncology, of the British Association of Cancer Research, of the European Association of Cancer Research, and of the Deutscher Krebskongress to find online published abstracts of their conferences. Data abstracted included study design, year of publication, country, matching used, percentage of response, exposure assessment (e.g., questionnaire, pharmacy database), frequency and duration of Aspirin use, total number of persons or person-years in each comparison group, outcome assessment, and relative risk with 95% confidence interval. We assumed that the OR from case-control studies provided a valid estimate for the relative risk. The estimators of the relative risk and related variances were abstracted, and were adjusted for the greatest number of covariates. If several exposure categories for the frequency and duration of Aspirin use had been published within one article, all of them were extracted. For each study, that exposure category which corresponded to the least common denominator of all studies was included in the meta-analysis.

7.7.3 Study Characteristics

A total of 15 studies (seven cohort studies and eight case-control studies) met the inclusion criteria. All studies were published in the English language. Estimates for the relative risk ranged from 0.71 to 1.12 within the prospective studies and from 0.4 to 1.13 within the retrospective studies. All but two studies compared Aspirin use with nonuse. One study defined nonexposure as Aspirin use shorter than 1 year and another study as Aspirin use less frequently than once per week. The definition of exposure was very heterogeneous and ranged from any use up to ten

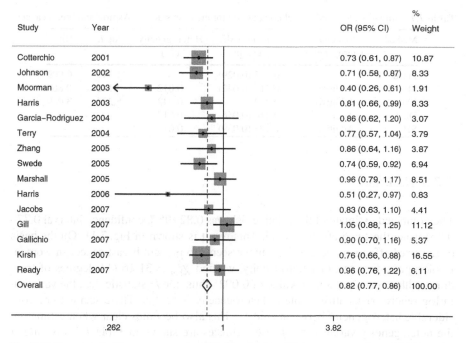

Fig. 7.11 Forest plot with summary estimate for the Aspirin and breast cancer data. *OR* odds ratio, *CI* confidence interval

different exposure categories. One study only gave information on the frequency of Aspirin use (Johnson et al. 2002), another presented estimates for both but not in combination (Garcia Rodriguez and Gonzalez-Perez 2004), and seven studies gave estimates for the combination of the duration and the frequency of Aspirin use (Cotterchio et al. 2001; Harris et al. 2005; Marshall et al. 2005; Swede et al. 2005; Terry et al. 2004; Zhang et al. 2005). The number of adjusted covariates ranged from one (Harris et al. 2003) to 17 (Zhang et al. 2005). Figure 7.11 shows the studies included sorted by year of publication.

7.7.4 Publication Bias

The regression model in which the estimated effect sizes were directly regressed on inverse variance as a predictor found no evidence of publication bias ($p = 0.87$). Furthermore, assessment of the funnel plot did not show strong patterns, although there were a few missing beyond an inverse variance of 40, which is an indicator for a lack of very small studies. Overall, the results did not reveal evidence for a substantial influence of publication bias.

Table 7.7 Estimates of τ^2 and model comparison for the case study of Aspirin and breast cancer

Method	Residual heterogeneity	Estimates (SE) intercept	Heterogeneity ($\hat{\tau}^2$)	$\log L$	BIC
Fixed	None	−0.205 (0.029)	–	1.349	0.009
Mixed	Additive	−0.213 (0.042)	0.012	3.142	−0.869
FM	Additive	−0.242	0.042	5.235	3.069
DL	Additive	−0.216 (0.046)	0.017	–	–
SH	Additive	−0.223 (0.059)	0.035	–	–

7.7.5 Results

The combined estimate of the relative risk was 0.82 (95% confidence interval 0.77–0.86) using the fixed effects model. This result is shown in Fig. 7.11. On the basis of the fixed effects model Aspirin intake seems to prevent breast cancer in women. Looking at a first test of heterogeneity, we find $\chi^2_{\text{het}} = 31.16$ (14 degrees of freedom) with a corresponding p value of 0.002. Thus, the I^2 statistic, i.e., the variation in log relative risks attributable to heterogeneity is 55.1%. There seems to be considerable heterogeneity between studies. This also becomes clear when estimating the heterogeneity variance τ^2. These estimates are shown in Table 7.7. Looking at the goodness-of-fit statistic BIC, at least the finite mixture model seems to provide a better fit than the homogenous model. The results of the mixture model are shown in Sect. 7.8.3.

The results of the heterogeneity analysis raise the question of whether known covariates explain at least some of the observed heterogeneity. This is considered in the next section.

7.7.6 Results of a Metaregression

In this metaregression we consider the covariates type of study (0 for case-control study, 1 for cohort study) and the year of publication centered on the year 2001. We start with the interpretation of the results in Table 7.8, looking first at the linear mixed model. In terms of the likelihood ratio test, the third mixed effects model with the covariates study type and year of publication provides the best fit to the data. The results of the metaregression provide several interesting insights. Looking at linear mixed effects models, the following comments are in order.

First, cohort studies provide less optimistic results than do case-control studies. In model 2 case-control studies estimate the mean OR of 0.74 cohort studies estimate a mean OR of $\exp(−0.305+0.187) = 0.89$. This is certainly less encouraging. Second, it is important to note that more recent studies provide less optimistic results than earlier studies. With each year from 2001 the OR on the log scale increases by 0.031 when adjustments are made for study type. Third, the covariates explain

Table 7.8 Metaregression for the Aspirin and breast cancer data

Type of model	Intercept	Type	Year	Heterogeneity (τ^2)	$\log L$	BIC
Fixed effects	−0.412	0.165	0.031	–	8.61	−9.09
	(0.078)	(0.071)	(0.016)			
Linear mixed effects 1	−0.213	–	–	0.012	3.14	−0.869
	(0.042)					
Linear mixed effects 2	−0.305	0.187	–	0.002	6.21	−4.375
Linear mixed effects 3	−0.412	0.165	0.031	0	8.61	−6.382
Finite mixture model						
Intercept 1 $\hat{p}_1 = 0.12$	−0.9154	0.079	0.034	0.03	10.53	−7.51
	(0.075)	(0.05)	(0.012)			
Intercept 2 $\hat{p}_2 = 0.87$	−0.357	–	–			
	(0.054)					

variability between studies. The estimate of τ^2 drops from 0.012 for the random effects model without covariates to zero when the covariates study type and year are included.

Now switching to the covariate-adjusted finite mixture model, we can still state an effect of study and year of publication. However, in contrast to the linear mixed effects model, the mixture model still identifies residual heterogeneity. Thirteen percent of the studies find a strong protective effect reflected by the intercept of that component equal to −0.92.

In terms of interpretation based on the linear mixed effects model the protective nature of Aspirin use seems questionable, whereas the mixture model seems to identify a subgroup with strong protective effects.

7.7.7 Modeling Dose Response

Investigation of a dose-response relationship is an important part in applying the criteria for a causal association in epidemiology (Hill 1965). Technically, the analysis of dose response may be seen as a special case of a meta-analysis or metaregression. In published studies which investigate a quantal relationship, most frequently the available information is given by the log relative risks ($\log RR_i$) at each dose level $x_{i\cdot} = 1, \ldots, m$. Dose response is then modeled by fitting a weighted least squares linear regression to the adjusted log (ORs) or relative risks (Greenland and Longnecker 1992):

$$\log RR_{ij} = \alpha_i + \beta_i x_{ij}, \tag{7.43}$$

where α_i is the intercept of the ith study, β_i is the corresponding slope of the ith study, and x_{ij} is the value of exposure in the jth exposure category.

One question to deal with is the use of the unexposed group. Following Smith et al. (1995), including the intercept α_i in the model results in the variable intercept model. This implies that the risk between two groups may differ before the initial dose. Forcing the intercept through zero is frequently called the zero intercept model. This implies that x_{ij} indicates exposure in the $j = 1, \ldots, J - 1$ nonreference categories.

In this case the model reduces to

$$\log RR_{ij} = \beta_i x_{ij} \, . \tag{7.44}$$

Most commonly $x_{ij} = 0$ is used as the reference category and by definition the log relative risk is zero in the reference category; thus, this model has no intercept. Hence, a meta-analysis of dose-response data may be undertaken using estimated regression coefficients $\hat{\beta}_i$ and corresponding standard errors $se(\hat{\beta}_i)$. Regression coefficients $\hat{\beta}_i$ may be obtained using a weighted linear regression with weights

$$w_{ij} = \frac{1}{\sigma_{ij}^2} \, . \tag{7.45}$$

Again, σ_i^2 is the variance of the jth relative risk or OR of the ith study. The slope standard error can be obtained as

$$se(\beta_i) = \frac{1}{\sum w_{ij} x_{ij}^2} \, . \tag{7.46}$$

Example Revisited

To investigate a dose-response relationship only studies could be included which reported information on the frequency and on the duration of Aspirin use. Studies which reported only the exposition category any use had to be excluded. We assigned scores to the categories of Aspirin intake. In the case of the category a to b, we chose the midpoint and in the case of the lowest categories $<a$, we assigned the score $a/2$. Since the score assignment for the upper, open-ended categories $(\geq a)$ most sensitively influences the estimated slope in categorical regression (Berlin et al. 1993; Il'yasova et al. 2005), Mangiapane et al. (2008) explored two approaches to assign a score to this category. If b_i represents the lower bound of the ith interval, where the intervals are indexed $i = 1, \ldots, n$, the first approach assigned the nth interval score as function of its lower bound multiplied by 1.233. Since Il'yasova et al. (2005) showed that more valid results can be obtained by using a function of the lower bound and the width of the previous interval, a second approach assigned the nth interval score as a function of $b_n + (b_n - b_{n-1})$. Scores were calculated for the frequency of use (pills per week) as well as for the duration of use. To combine frequency and duration of use, we calculated a combined variable (pill-years) by multiplying the number of pills per day and the number of years of Aspirin use. This leads to the combined variable pill-years (pills per day × years of use).

An initial analysis involves fitting model (7.44) to each study with sufficient data to combine frequency and duration into the variable pill-years. Table 7.9 shows the

Table 7.9 Aspirin and breast cancer: dose-response data

Study	Type	PPW	Duration	Pill-years	RR	95% CI	$\hat{\beta}$	SE($\hat{\beta}$)
Harris (2003)	Cohort	7	2.5	2.50	0.83	0.64–1.08		
		7	7	7.00	0.87	0.60–1.25	−0.022	(0.011)
		7	12	12.00	0.79	0.60–1.04		
Terry (2004)	Case control	3.5	2.5	1.25	1.13	0.64–1.99		
		8.4	2.5	3.00	0.74	0.54–1.01		
		3.5	6	3.00	0.89	0.64–1.24	−0.044	(0.019)
		8.4	6	7.20	0.77	0.57–1.04		
Jacobs (2005)	Cohort	9	2.5	3.21	1.08	0.94–1.23	−0.002	(0.013)
		9	6	7.71	0.88	0.69–1.12		
Swede (2005)	Case control	0.5	0.5	0.04	0.8	0.67–0.96		
		1	1.2	0.17	0.95	0.74–1.23		
		4	1.2	0.69	0.8	0.65–0.99		
		8.4	1.2	1.44	0.74	0.59–0.92		
		1.2	5	0.86	0.74	0.59–0.94	−0.040	(0.011)
		1.2	12	2.06	0.91	0.78–1.06		
		7	5	5.00	0.77	0.59–1.02		
		7	12	12.00	0.72	0.53–0.97		
Zhang (2005)	Case control	4.8	1	0.69	0.79	0.45–1.37		
		4.8	3	2.06	0.89	0.53–1.49		
		4.8	7	4.80	1.11	0.57–2.17	−0.023	(0.020)
		4.8	14.5	9.94	0.89	0.45–1.74		
		4.8	24	16.46	0.59	0.25–1.36		
Marshall (2005)	Cohort	3.5	2.5	1.25	1.05	0.87–1.25		
		3.5	6	3.00	1.12	0.99–1.26		
		7	2.5	2.50	1.00	0.84–1.2	0.011	(0.012)
		7	6	6.00	0.96	0.79–1.18		
Harris (2006)	Case control	2.5	5	1.79	1.02	0.3–3.57	−0.378	(0.11)
		4	5	2.86	0.39	0.22–0.72		
Ready (2007)	Cohort	2	1.5	2.14	0.76	0.55–1.05	0.035	(0.024)
		2	6	6.85	1.43	1.02–2.00		

PPW pills per week, *RR* relative risk, *CI* confidence interval, *SE* standard error

relative risk and ORs, respectively, for study-specific dose-response data together with the estimated regression coefficients.

The estimated regression coefficients $\hat{\beta}$ from Table 7.9 can now be subjected to meta-analysis as described within this chapter. That is, a weighted pooled estimate may be obtained together with a test for heterogeneity. Figure 7.12 shows a forest plot of the estimated regression coefficients together with their 95% confidence intervals.

Performing a fixed effects meta-analysis on the estimated slopes leads to an overall estimate of $\hat{\beta} = -0.02$ with a 95% confidence interval (-0.03 to -0.01). This indicates that there seems to be a dose-response relationship present and that with increasing dose the relative risk decreases. However, Fig. 7.12 shows substantial variability between studies. The variation among studies seems to be greater than the variation which can explained by the standard errors of the slopes. One way to address this problem would be to fit random effects models for the slopes as outlined by Dumouchel (1995).

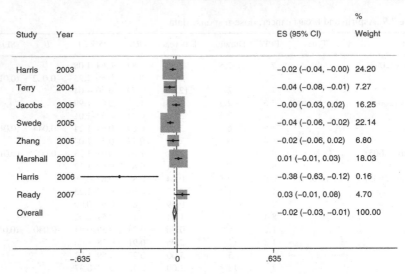

Fig. 7.12 Slope estimates (*ES*) and 95% confidence intervals for the Aspirin and breast cancer data

Instead of this two-step approach (first estimating regression coefficients and then performing a meta-analysis on these coefficients) here a one-step approach is proposed.

7.7.8 A Metaregression Model for Dose-Response Analysis

Consider fitting a zero-intercept model with random effects

$$\hat{\theta}_{ij} = \beta_1 x_{ij} + b_i x_{ij} + \varepsilon_i, \qquad b_i \sim N(0, \tau_1^2), \quad \varepsilon_i \sim N(0, \sigma_{ij}^2), \tag{7.47}$$

where $\hat{\theta}_{ij}$ are given by the $\log RR_{ij}$ of the respective studies and σ_{ij}^2 are the corresponding variances. As pointed out by Greenland and Longnecker (1992) the variance estimators of the regression coefficients β_i underestimate the true variance. This is due to the fact that using the same reference category for each exposure category induces a correlation which is ignored. Thus, Greenland and Longnecker (1992) estimated the covariance matrix based on the observed relative risks and the number of subjects in the respective exposure category. Often, these numbers are not available.

The application of a linear mixed effects model helps to account for the correlation within each study. To see this consider the intraclass correlation coefficient ρ_{is} in the ith study with dose levels x_{ij} and x_{is}. Then the respective variances and the covariance are given by

Table 7.10 Random effects dose-response regression

Model	Intercept (SE)	Slope (SE)	Heterogeneity (τ_1^2)	BIC
Zero intercept				
Fixed	–	−0.016 (0.005)	–	9.6
Random	–	−0.016 (0.009)	0.0003	6.3
Variable intercept				
Random	−0.071 (0.068)	−0.0089 (0.0086)	0.012	−8.5

$$\text{var}(\hat{\theta}_{ij}) = \tau_1^2 x_{ij}^2 + \sigma_{ij},$$

$$\text{var}(\hat{\theta}_{is}) = \tau_1^2 x_{is}^2 + \sigma_{is},$$

$$\text{cov}(\hat{\theta}_{ij}, \hat{\theta}_{is}) = \tau_1^2 x_{ij} x_{is}. \tag{7.48}$$

As a result, the intraclass correlation ρ_{is} is given by

$$\rho_{is} = \frac{\tau^2 x_{ij} x_{is}}{\sqrt{\tau_1^2 x_{ij}^2 + \sigma_{ij}} \sqrt{\tau_1^2 x_{is}^2 + \sigma_{is}}}. \tag{7.49}$$

Hence, this model is able to account for the induced correlation. Applying this model to our data, we obtain the results shown in Table 7.10. Calculating the likelihood ratio test for the models given in Table 7.10 leads to $6.2 - 2.1 = 4.1$. Thus, on the basis of the likelihood ratio statistic we would conclude that there is structural variability between the dose-response relationship in this meta-analysis. We would stick to the random effects model although the improvement looking at the BIC is not that strong. However, the more complex model also addresses the correlation within studies and is thus preferable. With the same argument we present only the random effects version of the model with variable intercepts.

Using the random effects model, the fixed effect of the variable "pill-years" is no longer statistically significant. As a result, there is no clear dose-response relationship when applying this model. The same applies if a model with variable intercepts is considered.

7.7.9 Discussion

At first sight this meta-analysis seems to support the hypothesis that Aspirin use has a protective effect with regard to breast cancer risk judging from the pooled relative risk of 0.82 (95% confidence interval 0.77, 0.86) based on the fixed effects model. However, this new meta-analysis of observational studies published between 2001 and 2007 does not provide a clear-cut protective association between Aspirin intake and breast cancer risk when a metaregression with covariates study type and year of publication based on a linear mixed effects model is performed. Cohort studies provide less optimistic results than case-control studies. Likewise, newer studies provide less support for a protective association. Additionally, the dose-response analysis neither using the variable-intercept model nor using the zero-intercept model provides substantial evidence of a clear-cut dose-response relationship.

However the metaregression based on the finite mixture with the same covariates still identifies residual heterogeneity and a subgroup with a strong protective effect. As a result, from the author's point of view it would be desirable to perform simulation studies for the estimation of the heterogeneity variance and covariate effects for metaregression.

7.8 Computation

7.8.1 "Standard Meta-analysis"

This section provides R and S-plus code which estimates the parameters of the various models. The dataframe containing the data for the meta-analysis and the metaregression is called "aspirin" and is part of the package CAMAN. In the beginning we start with the construction of a forest plot. A simple command is provided by the R library *rmeta* by Lumley (2008). In a first step a variable called "annotate" combining the name of the study and year of publication of the study is created. Then the function *metaplot* is used to build a forest plot on the log scale. The function takes as necessary arguments the effect sizes and corresponding standard errors. Additionally, we give the new variable "annotate."

```
> library(CAMAN)
> library(rmeta)
> data(aspirin)
> attach(aspirin)
> annotate<-cbind(name,year)
> metaplot(logrr,se,labels=annotate)
```

The result is shown in Fig. 7.13.

We continue with the fixed effects model. The standard fixed effects model can be fit using various R packages, e.g., *meta* by Schwarzer (2007). The function *metagen*, which has the log relative risks and corresponding standard errors as arguments, can be used to fit fixed effects and random effects models based on the DerSimonian–Laird approach. After installing the package and invoking the library, one uses the command *metagen*.

```
> library(meta)
> metagen(logrr,se)
```

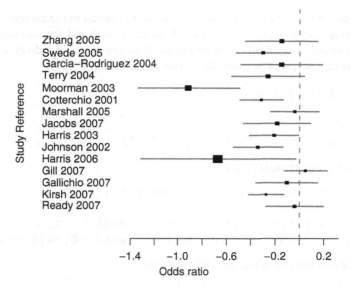

Fig. 7.13 Forest plot constructed with the function *metaplot*

This gives the shortened output

```
Number of trials combined: 15


Fixed effects model
                95%-CI              z      p.value
-0.2044   [-0.2630; -0.1459] -6.8478 < 0.0001
Random effects model
-0.2157   [-0.3078; -0.1235] -4.5883 < 0.0001

Quantifying heterogeneity:
tau^2 = 0.0168; H = 1.49 [1.12; 1.99];
    I^2 = 55.1% [19.6%; 74.9%]

Test of heterogeneity:
     Q d.f.  p.value
 31.16   14   0.0053
```

Various Estimates of the Heterogeneity Variance with the R/S-plus Function *mima*

The R/S-plus function *mima* (Viechtbauer 2006) may be used to obtain various estimates of the heterogeneity variance. To calculate the SH variance the following steps are required. For the very first use the function needs to be loaded with the *source* statement, which assumes that the function is stored in the current directory. Then an empty matrix of covariates needs to be created and the variances of the individual studies are calculated from the standard errors of the individual studies. Finally the function is called with the option *method = "SH"*

```
> source("mima.ssc")
> covar<- c()
> var<-se^2
> mima(logrr,var,covar,method="SH")
```

This gives the (shortened) output:

```
Estimate of (Residual) Heterogeneity: 0.0358

         estimate    SE     zval    pval    CI_L     CI_U
intrcpt   -0.2246  0.0597 -3.7596 2e-04 -0.3416 -0.1075
```

If the DL estimator is desired, the call is changed to

```
> mima(logrr,var,method="DL")
```

which gives the output

```
Estimate of (Residual) Heterogeneity: 0.0168
```

7.8.2 Meta-analysis with SAS

To the author's knowledge there are no specialized tools available to perform a meta-analysis in SAS; however, *proc mixed* may be used to perform maximum likelihood estimation.

```
data aspirin;
input name$  year logrr est type;
cards;
Cotterchio          2001     -0.31471    0.00820    0
Johnson             2002     -0.34249    0.01070    1
Moorman             2003     -0.91629    0.04672    0
Harris              2003     -0.21072    0.01070    1
Garcia-Rodriguez    2004     -0.15082    0.02906    0
Terry               2004     -0.26136    0.02353    0
Zhang               2005     -0.15082    0.02302    0
Swede               2005     -0.30111    0.01284    0
Marshall            2005     -0.04082    0.01048    1
Harris              2006     -0.67334    0.10749    0
Kirsh               2007     -0.27444    0.00539    0
Jacobs              2007     -0.18633    0.02022    1
Gill                2007      0.04879    0.00802    1
```

```
Gallichio              2007     -0.10536      0.01660      1
Ready                  2007     -0.04082      0.01458      1
;
run;
```

After the data have been read, some auxiliary variables are created in a data step, more precisely, weights $w_i = (1/\sigma_i^2)$, study number, and the centered variable year of publication are created:

```
data aspirin;
set aspirin;
study=_N_;
wgt=1./est;
yearc=year-2001;
run;
```

The study-specific variances σ_i^2 are fixed and known. In SAS terminology, we say that the R matrix for the residuals is known. There is no need to estimate the residual variance as long as we supply this information in the model and constrain R to be fixed at this value while estimating other parameters in the model. This requirement can be implemented through the *weight* and *parms* statements in the *mixed* procedure. A fixed effects model is then obtained by

```
proc mixed method=ml  data=aspirin;
class study;
weight wgt;
model logrr=  /s cl;
Parms  (1)/hold=(1);
run;
```

A random effects model is obtained with

```
proc mixed method=ml covtest cl data=aspirin;
class study;
weight wgt;
model logrr=  /s cl;
Random  int /type=un sub=study;
Parms (0.1)  (1)/hold=(2);
run;
```

Again, the study-specific variances are kept fixed; additionally a starting value for the heterogeneity variance is given.

7.8.3 Finite Mixture Models

A finite mixture model without covariates can be fit using the commands

```
> library(CAMAN)
> data(aspirin)
> mix.result<-mixalg(obs="logrr",var.lnOR="var",
                     data=aspirin)
```

This command expects the log relative risk and the corresponding variance. After running the combination of the VEM algorithm and the EM algorithm, one obtains the following result after typing *mix.result* on the command prompt:

```
> mix.result


      p            mean
1 0.07091158 -0.90089604
2 0.67435310 -0.25244617
3 0.25473532 -0.03451365

Log-Likelihood: 5.235441
BIC: 3.069368
```

Thus, the initial solution leads to a mixture of three components. This may be compared with a fixed effects model (one component only) using the EM algorithm.

This is achieved by typing

```
> m0<-mixalg.EM(mix.result,p=c(1),t=c(0))
```

This function expects the object of the previous analysis *mix0* and vectors of starting values for the mixing weights and component means, respectively.

This gives the result

```
> mix0


 p        mean
1 1 -0.2044453

Log-Likelihood: 1.349750
BIC: 0.008551024
```

To perform a forward selection, a solution with two components is obtained as follows:

```
 > m1<-mixalg.EM(mix.result,p=c(0.75,0.25),t=(-0.25,0))
```

or equivalently

```
 > m1<-mixalg.EM(obs="logrr",var.lnOR="var",
   p=c(0.75,0.25),t=c(-0.25,0),data=aspirin)
```

This gives the shortened result

```
> m1
          p          mean
1 0.7245986 -0.27411554
2 0.2754014 -0.03765404
```

```
Log-Likelihood: 3.794848    BIC: 0.5344549
```

To compare both models the function *anova* can be used. This function performs a parametric bootstrap to obtain the distribution of the likelihood ratio statistic.

```
> anova(m0,m1,nboot=2500)

   mixture model k        BIC        LL LL-ratio
1            m0 1 0.00914527 1.349452       NA
2            m1 2 0.53445492 3.794848 4.890791

LL ratios  bootstrap distribution'
     0.9      0.95     0.975       0.99
2.126616 3.633158 4.887770 6.546906
```

Judging from the likelihood ratio statistic, we reject the null hypothesis of a homogenous model, although the BIC is not considerably better.

7.8.4 Metaregression

Linear Mixed Effects Models with S-plus

Linear mixed effects models may be estimated using either SAS or S-plus, but unfortunately, to the author's knowledge, not with R. The reason for this is that the function *lme* of the package *nlme* does not handle fixed variances as needed. The following S-plus code computes the linear mixed effects model with covariates study type (0 for case-control study; 1 for cohort study) and year of publication centered on the year 2001.

```
> m2<-lme(fixed=logrr~type+yearc,data=aspirin,
  random=~1|study,
> weights=varFixed(~var),control=lmeControl(sigma=1),
  method="ML")
```

This gives the result

```
> m2

Linear mixed-effects model fit by maximum likelihood
  Data: aspirin
```

```
Log-likelihood: 8.607365
Fixed: logrr ~ type + yearc
(Intercept)          type        yearc
-0.4115349 0.1646794 0.03089528
```

```
Random effects:
 Formula:   ~ 1 | study
           (Intercept) Residual
StdDev: 0.0001318665          1
```

```
Variance function:
 Structure: fixed weights
 Formula:   ~ var
```

```
Number of Observations: 15
Number of Groups: 15
```

Linear Mixed Effects Models with SAS

Likewise, a random effects model with covariates study type and year of publication is obtained with the following code:

```
proc mixed method=ml covtest cl data=aspirin;
class study;
weight wgt;
model logrr= type yearc  /s cl;
Random  int /type=un sub=study;
Parms (0.1) (1)/hold=(2);
run;
```

Covariate-Adjusted Finite Mixture Models

The covariate-adjusted finite mixture model may be fit using the function *covmix*. The first entry gives the dependent variable "logrr." The second entry gives the variables for the fixed effects; the next entry gives the variables for the random effects. In this case none are given; this implies that different intercepts are fit. The next entry gives the dataframe to be used. Finally, the number of components is set to $k = 2$.

```
> mixcov(dep=c("logrr"),fixed=c("yearc","type"),
  random=c(""),data=aspirin,k=2)
```

This function gives the shortened output

```
Fit of the  2 -component mixture model:

coefficients:
               Estimate  Std. Error      t value        Pr(>|t|)
Z1          -0.915363239 0.074710396 -12.2521535 8.4297221e-16
Z2          -0.357015980 0.053778983  -6.6385781 7.7594519e-10
yearc        0.034441624 0.012115832   2.8426958 4.4353250e-04
typecohort   0.079095186 0.050181724   1.5761751 3.4666127e-02

 mixing weights:
  comp. 1   comp. 2
0.1333334 0.8666666

Log-Likelihood: 10.52891     BIC: -7.517567
```

Chapter 8
Analysis of Gene Expression Data

The analysis of gene expression data is a rapidly growing field of medical research. There is a large and increasing body of statistical literature on the analysis of microarray data. See, for example, the books by Parmigiani (2003), Simon et al. (2003), McLachlan et al. (2004), and Gentleman et al. (2005). Each human consists of a vast number of cells. With only a few exceptions, every cell of the body contains a full set of chromosomes contained in the *nucleus*. The human genome consists of 23 pairs of chromosomes which are the blueprint for all cellular activities. One pair of chromosomes is inherited from the father, the other one from the mother. Each chromosome consists of a chain of intertwined DNA, the double helix. Only small portions of DNA contain information for protein construction. These are called *genes*. "Gene expression" is the term used to describe the transcription of the information contained within the DNA into messenger RNA (mRNA), which is translated into proteins after a mRNA processing step. These perform most of the critical functions of cells. Thus, each gene specifies the composition and structure of proteins via mRNA. This gene expression is a complex and tightly regulated process that allows a cell to respond dynamically both to environmental stimuli and to its own needs.

8.1 DNA Microarrays

The great advancement of DNA microarrays is given by the fact that it is now possible to investigate simultaneously thousands of genes instead of looking at only a few. Technically speaking, DNA microarrays are small, solid supports containing the sequences of thousands of different genes attached at fixed locations. The supports themselves are usually glass microscope slides, but silicon chips and nylon membranes are used as well. The DNA is printed, spotted, or actually synthesized directly on the support. Gene sequences in a microarray are attached to their support in an orderly way, because the location of each spot in the array is used to identify a particular gene sequence. These spots are oligonucleotides consisting of fragments of DNA that are typically five to 50 nucleotides long.

P. Schlattmann, *Medical Applications of Finite Mixture Models*,
Statistics for Biology and Health, DOI: 10.1007/978-3-540-68651-4_8,
© Springer-Verlag Berlin Hiedelberg 2009

8.2 The Analysis of Differential Gene Expression

8.2.1 Analysis Based on Simultaneous Hypothesis Testing

Since the seminal paper of Golub et al. (1999), there has been considerable growth of the literature on analysis of gene expression and microarray data. At the beginning of microarray data analysis, research focused on clustering of genes and individuals on the basis of similar outcomes. In the terminology of statistical learning this is called *unsupervised learning*. Another approach involves the analysis of differentially expressed genes, that is, finding differences in gene expression levels between subgroups of individuals. For example, differences in gene expression between healthy tissue and tumor samples might be of interest. This is shown schematically in Fig. 8.1.

Statistical significance of differential gene expression can be tested by performing a hypothesis test for each of the m genes of the microarray, starting with a collection of null hypotheses

$$H_1, H_2, \ldots, H_m, \tag{8.1}$$

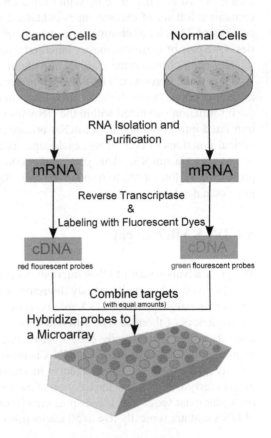

Fig. 8.1 A microarray. *mRNA* messenger RNA, *cDNA* complementary DNA

resulting in corresponding test statistics

$$T_1, T_2, \ldots, T_m \tag{8.2}$$

and their p values $P_1, P_2, \ldots, P_m$ which indicate how strongly the observed values t_i of the test statistics T_i contradict H_i, that is, $\Pr_{H_i}(|T_i| > |t_i|)$.

Assuming normality for the data and unequal variances, one such test would be the two-sample t test given by

$$t_i = \frac{\bar{x}_i - \bar{y}_i}{\sqrt{\frac{SD_{x_i}^2}{N} + \frac{SD_{y_i}^2}{M}}}, \quad i = 1, \ldots, m, \tag{8.3}$$

where $\bar{x}_i$ is the mean of the expression values $x_{i1}, \ldots, x_{iN}$ of the ith gene of the healthy tissues from $1, \ldots, N$ individuals. Likewise, $\bar{y}_i$ is the mean of measure of expression $y_{i1}, \ldots, y_{iM}$ from the of the ith gene from the tumor tissues of $1, \ldots, M$ individuals. Here, SD_x and SD_y denote the standard deviation of the respective groups. This test is then performed for each gene in the array.

The corresponding p value P_i of the respective test statistic is then obtained from

$$P_i = 1 - F_0(t_i) + F_0(-t_i), \tag{8.4}$$

where F_0 is the true distribution of the test statistic T_i under the null hypothesis.

To demonstrate the method, we apply data from the paper of Golub et al. dealing with patients suffering from leukemia. This is a famous and widely used data set. The author's interest was how could one use an initial collection of samples of bone marrow tissue belonging to known diagnostic categories such as acute myeloid leukemia (AML) and acute lymphatic leukemia (ALL) to distinguish those categories on the basis of microarray data. In our example we use both the training and the validation set of Golub et al. (1999) which consisted of 72 bone marrow samples (45 ALL, 27 AML) obtained from acute leukemia patients at the time of diagnosis. RNA prepared from bone marrow mononuclear cells was hybridized to high-density oligonucleotide microarrays, produced by Affymetrix, which contained probes for 7,129 human genes. Nowadays gene chips contain probes coding for up to 35,000 genes called "whole genome chips." A plot of the t test statistics and the corresponding p values is shown in Fig. 8.2. There are a total of 2,046 genes with a p value smaller than 0.05.

The main statistical problem in the analysis of microarray data is that the number m of genes is much larger than the number of samples. Thousands of genes are tested simultaneously. If, for example, a significance level of 0.01 is applied and 10,000 genes are tested, if no single gene is differentially expressed, we would expect $10,000 \times 0.01 = 100$ false-positive results. Multiple testing methods allow us to assess the statistical significance of findings. In the following, the notation of Benjamini and Hochberg (1995) for labeling correct and incorrect rejections is applied. When testing m hypotheses there are m_0 true null hypotheses and m_1 truly differentially expressed genes. The *observable* statistic R counts how many hypotheses

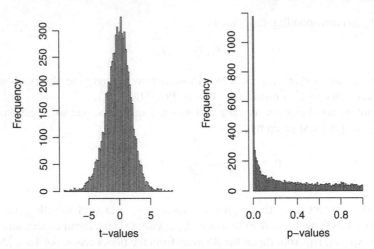

Fig. 8.2 Histogram of t statistics and corresponding p values of the data of Golub et al. (1999)

Table 8.1 Type I and Type II errors in multiple hypothesis testing

	No. of nonrejected hypotheses	No. of rejected hypotheses	Total
No. of true null hypotheses (non-differentially expressed genes)	U	V Type I error	m_0
No. of false hypotheses (differentially expressed genes)	T Type II error	S	m_1
Total	$m - R$	R	m

are rejected, that is, how many genes are called differentially expressed. Consequently V denotes the number of type I errors, i.e., false-positive results among the m tests. $S = R - V$ counts the number of correctly rejected hypotheses and T denotes the number of type II errors (false negatives). Table 8.1 gives an overview of the notation.

One approach to control the type I error rate is to control the *familywise error rate* (FWER). The FWER is defined as the probability of at least one type I error (false positive) among the genes selected as significant:

$$\text{FWER} = \Pr(V > 0). \qquad (8.5)$$

A famous procedure to control the FWER is the Bonferroni correction. Suppose that for each gene $i = 1, \ldots, m$ a hypothesis test is conducted. Then for each gene a test statistic T_i with corresponding unadjusted p value P_i is obtained. The Bonferroni adjusted p values are then given by

$$\tilde{P}_i = \min(mP_i, 1). \qquad (8.6)$$

Step 1: Rank the observed p values $P_{(1)} \leq P_{(2)} \leq, \ldots, \leq P_{(m)}$
Step 2: To control FDR= $E(V/R)$ at level α calculate

$$\hat{j} = \max_{1 \leq j \leq m} j : P_{(j)} \leq \frac{j}{m}\alpha$$

Step 3: If $\hat{j}$ exists, reject the null hypotheses corresponding to $P_{(1)} \leq P_{(2)} \leq, \ldots, \leq P_{r_{(\hat{j})}}$

Algorithm 8.2.1: Benjamini–Hochberg procedure to control the false discovery rate
(*FDR*)

Selecting all genes with $\tilde{P} \leq \alpha$ controls the FWER at level α, that is, $\Pr(V > 0) \leq \alpha$. In other words, the simplest Bonferroni procedure rejects those H_i for which $P_i \leq \alpha/m$. As a result, Bonferroni correction requires very small significance levels and leads to a loss of power. For our example 143 genes are selected when a Bonferroni corrected p value of 0.00000706 is applied. In this case we would conclude that there are 143 differentially expressed genes.

To obtain substantially more power the false discovery rate (FDR) may be used. In a seminal paper, Benjamini and Hochberg (1995) introduced the FDR as the expected proportion of type I errors (false positives) among the rejected hypotheses:

$$\text{FDR} = \text{E}(Q), \tag{8.7}$$

with

$$Q = \begin{cases} V/R, & \text{if } R > 0; \\ 0, & \text{if } R = 0. \end{cases} \tag{8.8}$$

One approach to controlling the FDR is to fix an acceptable FDR in advance and then to find a data-dependent threshold so that the FDR of this rule is less than or equal to the prechosen level. This was proposed by Benjamini and Hochberg (1995) and is referred as the BH procedure . The first step involves ranking the unadjusted p values. According to this step-down procedure the test of $H_{(1)}$ has p value $P_{(1)}$, the test of $H_{(2)}$ has p value $P_{(2)}$ and so forth. If $P_{(1)} > \alpha/m$, the BH procedure stops and no hypothesis is rejected. If $P_{(1)} \leq \alpha/m$, the procedure rejects $H_{(1)}$ and moves to $H_{(2)}$. Instead of comparing $P_{(2)}$ with α/m the BH procedure compares $P_{(2)}$ with $2\alpha/m$ and so on. This is the procedure given by Algorithm 8.2.1. Obviously this sequence of increasing thresholds has more power than a Bonferroni correction.

This rejection rule has

$$\text{FDR} \leq \alpha. \tag{8.9}$$

Inequality (8.9) becomes an equality when the p values P_i are independently and uniformly distributed. Obviously in gene expression studies dependence may occur. More recent articles have investigate the FDR under certain types of dependencies; see, for example, Benjamini and Yekutieli (2001) and Benjamini and Heller (2007).

Revisiting our example, we apply both a Bonferroni correction and the FDR to the data. Figure 8.3 compares the number of rejected hypotheses when no adjustment for multiple testing is performed, Bonferroni correction, and the approach based on

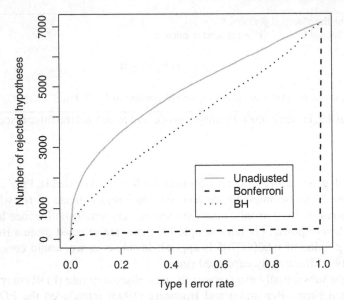

Fig. 8.3 Number of rejected hypothesis versus nominal type I error rate. *BH* Benjamini–Hochberg procedure

the FDR. Apparently, in this case the lowest number of rejections occurs when the FWER is controlled using the Bonferroni correction. The question arises whether this is always called for. One might argue that control of the FWER has to be chosen if high confidence in all selected genes is desired. This leads to a loss of power owing to the large number of tests. As a result, many differentially expressed genes may not appear significant.

On the other hand, if a certain proportion of false positives is tolerable, procedures based on the FDR are more flexible. In this case the researcher is free to select as many genes as practical considerations suggest.

In some cases even the unadjusted p values may be most appropriate, for example, if a comparison of functional categories of affected versus unaffected genes is desired.

8.2.2 A Mixture Model Approach

The problem of finding differentially expressed genes can be cast into a two-component mixture model framework. This idea was pursued by Lee et al. (2000), by Efron et al. (2001) and more recently by McLachlan et al. (2006).

The basic idea implies that a gene in the simplest case is either nondifferentially expressed or differentially expressed. Let p_0 be the probability that a gene is non-differentially expressed, p_1 be the probability that a gene is differentially expressed,

$f_0(w_i)$ be the density of a test statistic W of gene$_i$ which is nondifferentially expressed, and $f_1(w_i)$ be the density of a test statistic W of gene$_i$ which is differentially expressed. Then the marginal density for the ith gene is given by

$$f(w_i) = p_0 f_0(w_i) + (1 - p_0) f_1(w_i), \quad i = 1, \ldots, m. \tag{8.10}$$

Using Bayes's theorem, the posterior probability that the ith gene is nondifferentially expressed is given by

$$\tau_0(w_i) = \frac{p_0 f_0(w_i)}{p_0 f_0(w_i) + (1 - p_0) f_1(w_i)}. \tag{8.11}$$

Likewise, the posterior probability that the ith gene is differentially expressed is given by

$$\tau_1(w_i) = 1 - \frac{p_0 f_0(w_i)}{p_0 f_0(w_i) + (1 - p_0) f_1(w_i)}. \tag{8.12}$$

In this setting the gene-specific posterior probabilities provide the basis for statistical inference concerning differential expression. There is a close connection to the FDR method proposed by Benjamini and Hochberg (1995). It can be seen as an empirical Bayes version of the Benjamini and Hochberg (1995) method, using densities rather than tail areas. The posterior probability $\tau_0(w_i)$ was termed the "local false discovery rate" by Efron and Tibshirani (2002) and quantifies the gene-specific evidence for each gene.

It is obvious from (8.11) that to use this posterior probability of nondifferential expression in practice we need to be able to estimate p_0, the mixture density $f(w_i)$, and the null density $f_0(w_i)$. Efron et al. (2001) developed a simple empirical Bayes approach for this problem with minimal assumptions. This problem has been studied ever since under more specific assumptions by many authors see, for example, Newton et al. (2001), Newton et al. (2004), and Gottardo et al. (2006); Lo and Gottardo (2007).

Efron (2004) and McLachlan et al. (2006) propose working with z scores instead of p values P_i. Thus, we transform the p value P_i (whatever the test statistic) to a z score given by the following equation:

$$z_i = \Phi^{-1}(1 - P_i), \tag{8.13}$$

where $\Phi(\cdot)$ is the $N(0,1)$ standard normal cumulative distribution function. For example, $\Phi^{-1}(0.95) = 1.645$. This definition of z_i in (8.13) indicates that departures from the null are indicated by large positive values of z_i. If F_0 in (8.4) is the exact true null distribution, then z_i will have a standard normal distribution

$$z_i | H_i \sim N(0,1). \tag{8.14}$$

This is often called the *theoretical* null distribution.

Normal Mixture Model

Using z scores, one can cast the problem of finding differentially expressed genes into the framework of fitting a two-component mixture model of normals:

$$f(z_i) = p_0 N(z_i, 0, 1) + (1 - p_0) N(z_i, \mu, \sigma^2), \tag{8.15}$$

where $N(\cdot)$ denotes the normal density. Then $N(z_i, 0, 1)$ denotes the theoretical null and $N(z_i, \mu, \sigma^2)$ denotes the nonnull density of z_i, which is a normal density with mean μ and variance σ^2. For some microarray data sets the null distribution does not appear to be the standard normal distribution (Efron 2004). In this case the *empirical* null distribution needs to be estimated. To do this we replace the standard normal density $N(0, 1)$ by a normal density with mean μ_0 and variance σ^2. Also the assumption of a single component of differentially expressed genes can be relaxed. The nonnull distribution f_1 can be approximated by a mixture of k normal densities. Thus, combining the empirical null and an arbitrary number of components k, one can fit a normal mixture model to the data (z scores):

$$f(\hat{z}_i, P) = \sum_{j=1}^{k} p_j N(z_i, \mu_j, \sigma^2), \tag{8.16}$$

where again $N(\cdot)$ denotes the normal density. The parameters of the mixing distribution P are given by

$$P = \begin{bmatrix} \mu_1 & \cdots & \mu_k \\ p_1 & \cdots & p_k. \end{bmatrix}, \quad \text{with} \quad p_j \geq 0 \quad j = 1, \ldots, k, \tag{8.17}$$

$$p_1 + \cdots + p_k = 1. \tag{8.18}$$

These parameters need to be estimated from the data. The mixing weights p_j denote the a priori probability of an observation belonging to a certain subpopulation with parameter μ_j. Note that the number of components k needs to be estimated as well. This may again be done by combining the vertex exchange method and the expectation maximization (EM) algorithms outlined in Sect. 4.4.5.

Using the R package CAMAN, one can estimate the parameters of the model. See Table 8.2 for the results and Sect. 8.2.3 for a detailed description. This analysis leads to a mixture model with three components. About 61% of the genes are non-differentially expressed with $\hat{\pi}_0 = 0.61$ and a mean z score of 0.152. Note that the

Table 8.2 Finite mixture model for the data of Golub et al. (1999)

Component	Weights $\hat{p}$	Mean $\hat{\mu}$
1	0.610	0.152
2	0.343	1.817
3	0.047	3.964

empirical null differs from the theoretical null in this example. Another 34.5% of the genes show some evidence of differential expression (mean z score of 1.817). Another 4.7% of the genes are definitely differentially expressed with a mean z score of 3.964. On the basis of this approach the likelihood ratio statistic can be used as a formal test, whether differential gene expression is present or not. For the data at hand, a homogenous model leads to a log likelihood of $-12,874.2$, whereas the three-component mixture model shows a much larger log likelihood of $-12,757.12$. Thus, we would conclude that differential gene expression is present.

8.2.3 Computation

The following R code shows how to perform the calculations for the example using the data of Golub et al. (1999).

```
> data(golubMerge)
> idxALL <- which(sample.labels== "ALL")
> idxAML <- which(sample.labels == "AML")
```

The indicators "idxALL" and "idxAML" define the index of samples suffering from either ALL or AML, respectively. The gene expression data are then extracted from the gene expression data set.

In the next step the standard two-sample t test is applied to each of the 7,129 genes of the data set. The corresponding p values are stored in the variable *pvals*. This variable is then transformed to z scores.

```
> pvals <- apply(golubMerge.exprs, 1,
> function(x){t.test(x[idxAML],x[idxALL])[[3]]})
> zvals <- qnorm(1-pvals)
```

Now a mixture of normals is fit to the data, assuming a normal distribution for the z scores. Potential means are searched for on a grid with 25 grid points by applying the mixture algorithm described in Sect. 4.4.5. Here the empirical variance is automatically used as a fixed variance estimate for the normal density. This is the default for the function *mixalg*.

```
> mix <- mixalg.VEM(obs=zvals, family="gaussian",
startk=25)

> vem.gene<-mix@VEM_result
```

A plot of the grid points together with the mixing weights as shown in Fig. 8.4 is constructed using the standard R function *barplot*. From Fig. 8.4 there seem to be at least two classes of different gene expression.

```
>  barplot(vem.gene[,1],names=round(vem.gene[,2],2),
xlab="z-scores", ylab="Weights")
```

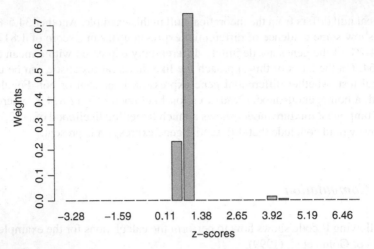

Fig. 8.4 Result of the vertex exchange method (VEM) algorithm for the 7,129 genes of the data of Golub et al. (1999)

The hybrid mixture algorithm continues then with the EM algorithm. Here the variance is updated in every EM iteration as defined in (4.43). This leads to a mixture model with three components. Typing *mix* shows the result of this model:

```
> mix
          p          mean
1 0.60919177 0.1523333
2 0.34319415 1.8162507
3 0.04761408 3.9643716

common variance: 1.09246943625579

Log-Likelihood: -12757.12      BIC: 25558.6
```

This result is then used to construct a histogram of the z scores together with the superimposed mixture model. The following code leads to Fig. 8.5:

```
hist(mix)
```

8.3 A Change of Perspective: Applying Methods from Meta-analysis

In the previous section differentially expressed genes where identified using hypothesis tests. The problem of multiplicity was addressed either by controlling the FWER using Bonferroni correction or by applying the BH procedure. To circumvent the problem of multiplicity, the problem was cast into a finite mixture model

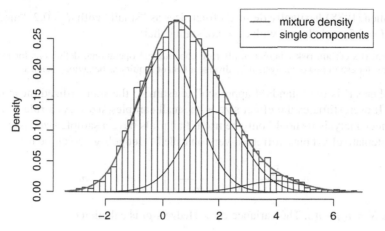

Fig. 8.5 Histogram of z scores and superimposed mixture model for the data of Golub et al. (1999)

framework using mixtures of normals by transforming p values into z scores. In this section it is proposed to change the perspective from considering hypothesis tests $H_1, H_2, \ldots, H_m$ that specify values for parameters $\theta_1, \theta_2, \ldots, \theta_m$ with null hypotheses $H_i : \theta_i = 0$ to effect sizes θ_i. This leads to the application of the meta-analytic methods described in Chap. 7 to the analysis of microarray data.

In order to apply meta-analytic methods the standardized mean difference, also known as Cohen's d, is calculated for each gene:

$$d_i = \frac{\bar{x}_i - \bar{y}_i}{s_i}, \quad i = 1, \ldots, m, \tag{8.19}$$

where again $\bar{x}_i$ is the mean of the ith sample $x_{i1}, \ldots, x_{in_x}$ from the m genes of the healthy tissues from $1, \ldots, n_x$ individuals and $\bar{y}_i$ is the mean of the sample $y_{i1}, \ldots, y_{in_y}$ from the m genes from the tumor tissues of $1, \ldots, n_y$ individuals. In other words, calculating Cohen's d implies standardizing the mean fold change $\bar{x}_i - \bar{y}_i$ with the pooled standard deviation s_i of each gene (study):

$$s_i = \sqrt{\frac{(n_{xi} - 1)\mathrm{SD}_{xi}^2 + (n_{yi} - 1)\mathrm{SD}_{yi}^2}{n_{xi} + n_{yi} - 2}}, \quad i = 1, \ldots, m, \tag{8.20}$$

where SD_{xi} and SD_{yi} denote the standard deviation of the respective groups in the ith sample. In the next step the variance σ_i^2 of Cohen's d_i is calculated as

$$\sigma_i^2 = \frac{n_{xi} + n_{yi}}{n_{xi} n_{yi}} + \frac{d_i^2}{2(n_{xi} + n_{yi} - 2)}. \tag{8.21}$$

In principle n_x and n_y would be expected to be constant for each gene. However, missing values occur. This is one reason to index sample sizes n_x and n_y. The other reason is to use standard notation from the meta-analytic literature.

Cohen (1988) hesitantly defined effect sizes as "small" with $d = 0.2$, "medium" with $d = 0.5$, and "large" with $d = 0.8$, stating that:

There is a certain risk inherent in offering conventional operational definitions for those terms for use in power analysis in as diverse a field of inquiry as behavioral science (p. 25).

Cohen's d is the "standard approach" to estimate the standardized mean difference. It overestimates the effect size with small samples sizes. As a rule of thumb in a meta-analysis it should only be used if all trials have a sample size greater than 10. Alternatively, a bias-corrected version called "Hedge's g" could be used:

$$g_i = \frac{\bar{x}_i - \bar{y}_i}{s_i} \left(1 - \frac{3}{4N_i - 9} \right), \quad i = 1, \dots, m, \tag{8.22}$$

where $N_i = n_{xi} + n_{yi}$. The variance σ_i of Hedge's g_i is calculated as

$$\sigma_i^2 = \frac{N_i}{n_{xi} n_{yi}} + \frac{g_i^2}{2(N_i - 3.94)}. \tag{8.23}$$

Now applying either Cohen's d or Hedge's g, we are in are in a situation where we have an effect size θ with corresponding variance σ_i^2. In contrast to many meta-analyses summarizing the evidence from the published literature, the interest here is in identifying differentially expressed genes. This leads immediately to the need to perform an analysis of heterogeneity, which may be done using a finite mixture model.

Again, we suppose that the gene-specific estimators $\hat{\theta}_1, \hat{\theta}_2, \dots, \hat{\theta}_m$ come from k subpopulations θ_j, $j = 1, \dots, k$. Assuming normality for the effect of each gene,

$$f(\hat{\theta}_i, \theta_j) = \frac{1}{\sqrt{2\pi\sigma_i^2}} \exp\left[-\frac{(\hat{\theta}_i - \theta_j)^2}{2\sigma_i^2} \right], \quad j = 1, \dots, q, \tag{8.24}$$

This leads to a finite mixture model with

$$f(\hat{\theta}_i, P) = \sum_{j=1}^{k} p_j f(\hat{\theta}_i, \theta_j, \sigma_i^2). \tag{8.25}$$

In this setting it is interesting to identify differentially expressed genes by calculating their posterior probability of component membership Z_{ij}. Applying Bayes's theorem and using the estimated mixing distribution as a prior distribution, we are able to compute the probability of each region belonging to a certain component, which is given by

$$\tau_{ij} = 1 \mid \hat{\theta}_i \hat{P}, \sigma_i^2 = \frac{\hat{p}_j f(\theta_i, \hat{\lambda}_j, E_i)}{\sum_{l=1}^{k} \hat{p}_l f(o_i, \hat{\lambda}_l, E_i)}. \tag{8.26}$$

The ith gene is then assigned to that subpopulation j for which it has the highest posterior probability τ_{ij} of belonging.

8.4 Case Study: Identification of a Gene Signature for Breast Cancer Prognosis

8.4.1 Introduction

It is well known that breast cancer patients with the same stage of disease can have markedly different treatment responses and overall outcome. The strongest predictors for metastases such as lymph node status and histologic grade often fail to classify breast tumors according to their clinical behavior. This led to a new line of research which aims to individualize therapy on the basis of the analysis of gene expression of the tumor cells; for an overview see, for example, van't Veer et al. (2005) and Brennan et al. (2007). The basic idea is to identify patients with tumor cells with a "good" signature who are likely to have a good prognosis and to identify patients with a "poor" signature whose prognosis is worse and who might benefit from adjuvant therapy. This is shown schematically in Fig. 8.6.

To this aim van't Veer et al. (2002) used DNA microarray analysis supervised classification to identify a gene expression signature strongly predictive of a short interval to distant metastases ("poor prognosis" signature) in patients without tumor cells in local lymph nodes at diagnosis, that is, lymph-node-negative patients. More

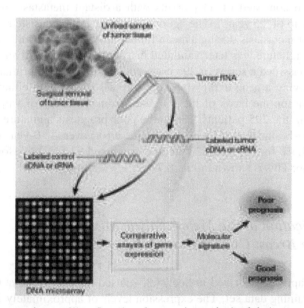

Fig. 8.6 Gene expression profiling. Samples of tumor tissue obtained during surgery are the material for gene expression profiling. Expression levels of a set of prognostically relevant genes are determined by DNA microarray analysis. On the basis of these molecular signatures patients are classified into groups with a poor or a good prognosis. (Reprinted with permission from Sauter and Simon (2002). Copyright 2002 Massachusetts Medical Society)

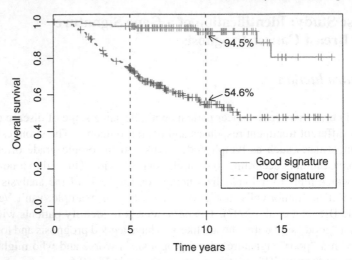

Fig. 8.7 Prognosis of breast cancer patients: "good" versus "poor" signature according to the study of van de Vijver et al. (2002)

precisely, employing univariate ranking of the genes and supervised classification led to a signature profile of 70 genes predictive of disease outcome. The "poor"-outcome group consisted of 34 patients with a distant metastasis within 5 years (mean follow-up of 2.5 years). The "good"-outcome group consisted of 44 patients with no distant metastasis during a mean follow-up of 8.7 years (minimum 5 years).

This gene signature was later validated in a study by van de Vijver et al. (2002). The authors classified a series of 295 consecutive patients with primary breast carcinomas as having a gene expression signature associated with either a poor or a good prognosis on the basis of the 70 genes from the study of van't Veer et al. (2002). Among the 295 patients, 180 had a poor-prognosis signature and 115 had a good-prognosis signature. Mean ($\pm$standardc error) overall 10-year survival rates were $54.6 \pm 4.4\%$ for the "good"-outcome group and $94.5 \pm 2.6\%$ for the "poor"-outcome group. This is shown in Fig. 8.7.

8.4.2 Application of the Meta-analytic Mixture Model to the Breast Cancer Data

To apply the approach derived in Sect. 8.3 we used the data from van't Veer et al. (2002) as a training data set. The expression levels of approximately 25,548 genes were available for the study consisting of 78 patients. For all of these genes the log mean ratio of the intensities of the red and green channels was used. This reflects the extent of induction or repression of a given gene. Note that we did not perform a preselection of genes. Like Bair and Tibshirani (2004) we used the total of 25,548 genes to develop our model.

Table 8.3 Data of van't Veer et al. (2002): result of the mixture model

Component	Weights $\hat{p}_j$	Standardized effect sizes $\hat{\theta}_j$
1	0.002	−0.570
2	0.442	−0.157
3	0.411	0.124
4	0.131	0.169
5	0.014	0.299

Now calculating for each gene Cohen's d_i with corresponding variance σ_i^2 allows us to treat the data as an analysis of heterogeneity within a meta-analysis. The first step involves estimating the parameters of the finite mixture model given by (8.25). Using Algorithm 4.4.5 within the R package CAMAN leads to the result in Table 8.3. Here a solution consisting of five mixture components is found. In terms of the magnitude of the effect, the first and the fifth components are notable. The first component has a mean effect size $\hat{\theta}_1 = -0.570$ with corresponding weight $\hat{p}_1 = 0.002$. This may be called a medium effect size. For the fifth component, we have a mean standardized effect size $\hat{\theta}_5 = 0.299$ with mixing weight $\hat{p}_5 = 0.014$.

To identify potentially predictive genes the posterior probability τ_{ij} is calculated as defined in (8.26) and the individual gene is categorized using a maximum rule. This leads to the selection of 30 genes with potential predictive power. Eight of these genes belong to the 70 genes which form the gene expression profile of van't Veer et al. (2002).

8.4.3 Validation of Results

The above-mentioned selected 30 genes were then applied to the data from the validation study of van de Vijver et al. (2002). This study comprised 295 women with breast cancer. Tumor tissues were selected from the fresh-frozen-tissue bank of the Netherlands Cancer Institute. The women were selected if the primary invasive breast carcinoma had a diameter less than 5 cm. The age at diagnosis was 52 years or younger and the year of diagnosis was between 1984 and 1995. Finally there was no previous history of cancer, except nonmelanoma skin cancer. All patients had been treated by modified radical mastectomy or breast-conserving surgery, including dissection of the axillary lymph nodes. The 78 patients used to build the model in the original study were included in the larger data set of 295 patients.

The 30 genes were used to build a prognostic index P_I given by

$$P_I = X\hat{\beta}. \tag{8.27}$$

Here the matrix X denotes the design matrix with dimension 295×30 and $\hat{\beta}$ denotes the vector of estimated ridge regression coefficients obtained by using a Cox regression with the end point overall survival. Figure 8.8 shows the prognosis of patients based on the median split prognostic index.

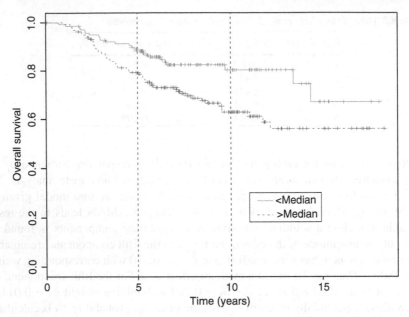

Fig. 8.8 Prognosis of breast cancer patients based on the prognostic index derived by the mixture model

Table 8.4 Comparison of the values of the R^2 statistic of the Cox proportional hazards model obtained by fitting the times of death to the mixture-derived prognostic indices and the discrete predictor described in van't Veer et al. (2002)

Method	No. of genes	R^2
Mixture model	8	0.142
Mixture model	30	0.201
Method of van't Veer et al. (2002)	70	0.120

To evaluate the predictive performance of the respective methods a Cox proportional hazards model was fit to each predictor. For each model the R^2 statistic was computed. R^2 measures the percentage of the variation in survival time that is explained by the model. As a result, when comparing models, one would prefer the model with the larger R^2 statistic (Table 8.4). Apparently the mixture approach based on either eight or 30 genes produced a stronger predictor of survival than the procedure described in van't Veer et al. (2002). Furthermore, our method used only eight or 30 genes, whereas the predictor of van't Veer et al. (2002) used 70 genes. Utilization of fewer genes results in a higher predictive power for this data set. This was also found by Bair and Tibshirani (2004), who applied their method of supervised principal components to the data. They applied five genes which were in common with the 70 genes of van't Veer et al. (2002). Jiang and Zhao (2006) discovered 13 genes as the most informative ones to predict the clinical outcomes of breast cancer patients with lymph-node-negative status. van Houwelingen et al.

(2006) applied cross-validated proportional hazards ridge regression to a subset of 4,096 genes of the said data set. This diversity of methods indicates the lack of standards and the need for further research.

From the medical point of view as pointed out by Bueno-de Mesquita et al. (2007) future studies should assess whether use of the prognosis signature could improve survival or equal survival while avoiding unnecessary adjuvant systemic treatment without affecting patients' survival. Additionally, studies are needed which assess the factors that physicians use to recommend adjuvant systemic treatment.

References

Agha, M. and D. Branker (1997). Algorithm AS 317: Maximum likelihood estimation and goodness-of-fit tests for mixtures of distributions. *J. R. Stat. Soc., Ser. C 46*(3), 399–407.

Agha, M. and M. Ibrahim (1984). Maximum likelihood estimation of mixtures of distribution. *J. R. Stat. Soc., Ser. C 33*, 327–332.

Ahrens, W. and I. Pigeot (Eds.) (2007). *Handbook of Epidemiology. Corrected 2nd printing.* Berlin: Springer. xi, 1617 p.

Ainsworth, L. M. and C. B. Dean (2006). Approximate inference for disease mapping. *Computational Statistics and Data Analysis 50*(10), 2552–2570.

Aitkin, M., D. Anderson, and J. Hinde (1981). Statistical modelling of data on teaching styles (with discussion). *J. R. Statist. Soc. A 144*, 419–461.

Aitkin, M., B. Francis, and J. Hinde (2006). *Statistical Modelling in GLIM 4* (Second ed.). Oxford: Oxford University Press.

Aitkin, M. and D. B. Rubin (1985). Estimation and hypothesis testing in finite mixture models. *J. R. Stat. Soc., Ser. B 47*, 67–75.

Aitkin, M. and G. T. Wilson (1980). Mixture models, outliers, and the EM algorithm. *Technometrics 22*, 325–331.

Ajith, T. and M. Soja (2006). A comparative study on the antimutagenicity of atorvastatin and lovastatin against directly acting mutagens. *Cell Biol Toxicol 22*(4), 269–74.

Ajith, T., J. Subin, J. Jacob, P. Sanjay, and N. Babitha (2005). Antimutagenic and anti-oxidant activities of the non-steroidal anti-inflammatory drug celecoxib. *Clin Exp Pharmacol Physiol 32*(10), 888–93.

Alexander, F., P. Boyle, P. Carli, J. Coebergh, G. Draper, A. Ekbom, F. Levi, P. McKinney, W. McWhirter, J. Michaelis, R. Peris-Bonet, E. Petridou, V. Pompe-Kirn, I. Plisko, E. Pukkala, M. Rahu, H. Storm, B. Terracini, L. Vatten, and N. Wray (1998). Spatial clustering of childhood leukaemia: summary results from the EUROCLUS project. *Br J Cancer 77*(5), 818–24.

Allam, M., A. Del Castillo, and R. Navajas (2003). Parkinson's disease, smoking and family history: meta-analysis. *Eur J Neurol. 10*, 59–62.

Ames, B., J. McCann, and E. Yamasaki (1975a). Methods for detecting carcinogens and mutagens with the Salmonella/mammalian-microsome mutagenicity test. *Mutat Res 31*(6), 347–64.

Ames, B., J. McCann, and E. Yamasaki (1975b). Proceedings: carcinogens are mutagens: a simple test system. *Mutat Res 33*(1 Spec No), 27–8.

Arcidiacono, P. and J. Jones (2003). Finite mixture distributions, sequential likelihood and the EM algorithm. *Econometrika 71*(3), 933–946.

Arun, B. and P. Goss (2004, Apr). The role of cox-2 inhibition in breast cancer treatment and prevention. *Semin.Oncol. 31*, 22–29.

Atwood, L., A. Wilson, J. Bailey-Wilson, J. Carruth, and R. Elston (1996). On the distribution of the likelihood ratio test statistic for a mixture of two normal distributions. *Commun. Stat., Simulation Comput. 25*(3), 733–740.

Bair, E. and R. Tibshirani (2004). Semi-supervised methods to predict patient survival from gene expression data. *PLoS Biol 2*(4), E108.

Bates, D. and D. Watts (1988). *Nonlinear regression analysis and its applications.* Wiley Series in Probability and Mathematical Statistics. New York etc.: John Wiley & Sons.

Becker, N., R. Frentzel-Beyme, and G. Wagner (1984). *Atlas of Cancer Mortality in the Federal Republic of Germany.* Springer, Berlin.

Begg, C. and M. Mazumdar (1994). Operating characteristics of a rank correlation test for publication bias. *Biometrics. 50*, 1088–101.

Bellec, S., D. Hemon, J. Rudant, A. Goubin, and J. Clavel (2006). Spatial and space-time clustering of childhood acute leukaemia in France from 1990 to 2000: a nationwide study. *Br J Cancer 94*(5), 763–70.

Benjamini, Y. and R. Heller (2007). False discovery rates for spatial signals. *Journal of the American Statistical Association 102*(480), 1272–1281.

Benjamini, Y. and Y. Hochberg (1995). Controlling the false discovery rate - a practical and powerful approach to multiple testing. *Journal of the Royal Statistical Society Series B-Methodological 57*(1), 289–300.

Benjamini, Y. and D. Yekutieli (2001). The control of the false discovery rate in multiple testing under dependency. *Annals of Statistics 29*(4), 1165–1188.

Bennett, D. (2003). Review of analytical methods for prospective cohort studies using time to event data: single studies and implications for meta-analysis. *Statistical Methods in Medical Research 12*, 297–319.

Berchtold, A. (2004). Optimization of mixture models: Comparison of different strategies. *Computational Statistics 19*(3), 385–406.

Berkey, C., D. Hoaglin, F. Mosteller, and G. Colditz (1995). A random-effects regression model for meta-analysis. *Stat Med 14*(4), 395–411.

Berlin, J. (1995). Invited commentary: Benefits of heterogeneity in meta-analysis of data from epidemiologic studies. *Am J Epidemiol 142*, 383–387.

Berlin, J., C. Begg, and T. Louis (1989). An assessment of publikation bias using a sample of published clinical trials. *Journal of the American Statistical Association 84*, 381–392.

Berlin, J. A., M. P. Longnecker, and S. Greenland (1993, May). Meta-analysis of epidemiologic dose-response data. *Epidemiology 4*, 218–228.

Bertz, R. and G. Granneman (1997). Use of in vitro and in vivo data to estimate the likelihood of metabolic pharmacokinetic interactions. *Clin Pharmacokinet 32*(3), 210–58.

Besag, J. and J. Newell (1991). The detection of clusters in rare diseases. *Journal of the Royal Statistical Society, Series A 154*, 143–156.

Besag, J., J. York, and A. Mollie (1991). Bayesian image restoration with two applications in spatial statistics. *Annals of the Institute of Statistical Mathematics 43*, 1–59.

Biernacki, C. (2004). Initializing EM using the properties of its trajectories in Gaussian mixtures. *Statistics and Computing 14*(3), 267–279.

Biernacki, C., G. Celeux, and G. Govaert (2003). Choosing starting values for the EM algorithm for getting the highest likelihood in multivariate Gaussian mixture models. *Computational Statistics and Data Analysis 41*(3-4), 561–575.

Biernacki, C., G. Celeux, G. Govaert, and F. Langrognet (2006, NOV 15). Model-based cluster and discriminant analysis with the MIXMOD software. *Computational Statistics and Data Analysis 51*(2), 587–600.

Bithell, J. (2001). Childhood leukaemia clustering–fact or artefact? *Methods Inf Med. 40*, 127–131.

Bithell, J. (2007). *Geographical Epidemiology*, pp. 861–890. In Ahrens and Pigeot Ahrens and Pigeot (2007).

Bithell, J. and R. Stone (1989). On statistical methods for analysing the geographical distribution of cancer cases near nuclear installations. *J Epidemiol Community Health 43*(1), 79–85.

Bjelakovic, G., D. Nikolova, L. Gluud, R. Simonetti, and C. Gluud (2007). Mortality in randomized trials of antioxidant supplements for primary and secondary prevention: systematic review and meta-analysis. *JAMA 297*(8), 842–57.

Black, D. (1984). Investigation of the possible increased incidence of cancer in West Cumbria. Report of the Independent Advisory Group. Technical report, HMSO.

Blettner, M., W. Sauerbrei, B. Schlehofer, T. Scheuchenpflug, and C. Friedenreich (1999). Traditional reviews, meta-analyses and pooled analyses in epidemiology. *Int J Epidemiol 28*, 1–9.

Blettner, M. and P. Schlattmann (2007). *Meta-Analysis in Epidemiology*, pp. 829–859. In Ahrens and Pigeot (2007).

Bloomfield, P. (1973). An exponential model for the spectrum of a scalar time series. *Biometrika 60*, 217–226.

Bloomfield, P. (2000). *Fourier analysis of time series. An introduction.* 2nd ed. Wiley Series in Probability and Mathematical Statistics. Applied Probability and Statistics. Chichester: Wiley. xiv, 261 p.

Boeckmann, A., L. Sheiner, and S. Beal (1994). *NONMEM Users Guide: Part V.* NONMEM Project Group University of California, San Francisco.

Böhning, D. (1982). Convergence of Simar's algorithm for finding the maximum likelihood estimate of a compound Poisson process. *Ann. Stat. 10*, 1006–1008.

Böhning, D. (1994). A note on a test for Poisson overdispersion. *Biometrika 81*(2), 418–419.

Böhning, D. (1995). A review of reliable maximum likelihood algorithms for semiparametric mixture models. *J. Stat. Plann. Inference 47*(1-2), 5–28.

Böhning, D. (1999a). *C.A.MAN-Computer Assisted Analysis of Mixtures and Applications.* Chapman and Hall.

Böhning, D. (1999b). *Computer-Assisted Ananlysis of Mixtures and Applications: Meta-Analysis, Disease Mapping and Others.* Boca Raton, Florida: Boca Raton: Chapman & Hall/CRC.

Böhning, D. (2003). The EM algorithm with gradient function update for discrete mixtures with known (fixed) number of components. *Statistics and Computing 13*(3), 257–265.

Böhning, D., E. Dietz, R. Schaub, P. Schlattmann, and B. G. Lindsay (1994). The distribution of the likelihood ratio for mixtures of densities from the one-parameter exponential family. *Ann. Inst. Stat. Math. 46*(2), 373–388.

Böhning, D., E. Dietz, and P. Schlattmann (1998). Recent developments in computer assisted mixture analysis. *Biometrics 54*, 283–303.

Böhning, D., U. Malzahn, E. Dietz, P. Schlattmann, C. Viwatwongkasem, and A. Biggeri (2002). Some general points in estimating heterogeneity variance with the DerSimonian-Laird estimator. *Biostatistics. 3*, 445–57.

Böhning, D. and P. Schlattmann (1999). Disease mapping with a hidden structure using mixture models. In A. Lawson, A. Biggeri, D. Böhning, E. Lesaffre, J. F. Viel, and R. Bertollini (Eds.), *Disease Mapping and Risk Assessment for Public Health decision making.* Wiley, Chichester.

Böhning, D., P. Schlattmann, and B. G. Lindsay (1992). C.A.MAN- computer assisted analysis of mixtures: Statistical algorithms. *Biometrics 48*, 283–303.

Boos, D. D. (1992). On Generalized Score Tests. *The American Statistician 46*(4), 327–333.

Box, G. (1979). *Robustness in the strategy of scientific model building*, pp. 202–236. Academic Press, New York.

Boyd, N., L. Martin, M. Noffel, G. Lockwood, and D. Trichler (1993). A meta-analysis of studies of dietary fat and breast cancer. *Br J Cancer 68*, 627–636.

Boyd, S. and L. Vandenberghe (2004). *Convex optimization.* Cambridge University Press. xiii, 716 p.

Breast Cancer, C. C. G. O. H. F. (1996). Breast cancer and hormonal contraceptives: collaborative reanalysis of individual data on 53 297 women with breast cancer and 100 239 women without breast cancer from 54 epidemiological studies. *Lancet 347*, 1713–1727.

Brennan, D., C. Kelly, E. Rexhepaj, P. Dervan, M. Duffy, and W. Gallagher (2007). Contribution of DNA and tissue microarray technology to the identification and validation of biomarkers and personalised medicine in breast cancer. *Cancer Genomics Proteomics 4*(3), 121–34.

Breslow, N. (1984). Extra-poisson variation in log-linear models. *Applied Statistics-Journal of the Royal Statistical Society Series C 33*(1), 38–44.

Breslow, N. (1990). Test of Hypotheses in Overdispersed Poison regression. *Journal of the American Statistical Association 85*(410), 565–571.

Breslow, N. and N. Day (1987). *Statistical Methods in Cancer Research, Volume II -The Design and Analysis of Cohort Studies.* IARC Scientific publications No. 82.

Bretz, F. and L. Hothorn (2003). Statistical analysis of monotone or non-monotone dose-response data from in vitro toxicological assays. *Altern Lab Anim 31 Suppl 1*, 81–96.

Brillinger, D. R. (2001). *Time series. Data analysis and theory. Repr.* Classics in Applied Mathematics. 36. Philadelphia, PA: SIAM. xx, 540 p.

Brockwell, S. and I. Gordon (2001). A comparison of statistical methods for meta-analysis. *Stat Med 20*(6), 825–40.

Bueno-de Mesquita, J. M., W. H. van Harten, V. P. Retel, L. J. van't Veer, F. S. van Dam, K. Karsenberg, K. F. Douma, H. van Tinteren, J. L. Peterse, J. Wesseling, T. S. Wu, D. Atsma, E. J. Rutgers, G. Brink, A. N. Floore, A. M. Glas, R. M. Roumen, F. E. Bellot, C. van Krimpen, S. Rodenhuis, M. J. van de Vijver, and S. C. Linn (2007). Use of 70-gene signature to predict prognosis of patients with node-negative breast cancer: a prospective community-based feasibility study (RASTER). *Lancet Oncol 8*(12), 1079–87.

Bustad, A., D. Terziivanov, R. Leary, R. Port, A. Schumitzky, and R. Jelliffe (2006). Parametric and nonparametric population methods - Their comparative performance in analysing a clinical dataset and two Monte Carlo simulation studies. *Clinical Pharmacokinetics 45*(4), 365–383.

Cameron, A. and P. Trivedi (1998). *Regression analysis of count data.* Cambridge University press.

Cameron, M. A. and T. Turner (1987). Fitting models to spectra using regression packages. *J. R. Stat. Soc., Ser. C 36*, 47–57.

Caraballoso, M., M. Sacristan, C. Serra, and X. Bonfill (2003). Drugs for preventing lung cancer in healthy people. *Cochrane Database Syst Rev* (2), CD002141.

Carlin, B. and T. A. Louis (1996). *Bayes and empirical Bayes methods for data analysis.* Monographs on Statistics and Applied Probability. 69. London: Chapman and Hall.

Cawello, W. (Ed.) (1999). *Parameters for Compartment-free Pharmacokinetics - Standardisation of Study Design, Data Analysis and Reporting.* Aachen, Germany: Shaker Verlag.

Celeux, G., D. Chauveau, and J. Diebolt (1996). Stochastic versions of the EM algorithm: An experimental study in the mixture case. *Journal of Statisitcal Computaton and Simulation 55*(4), 287–314.

Chatfield, C. (2004). *The analysis of time series* (Sixth ed.). Chapman and Hall/CRC, Boca Raton.

Chen, H., J. Chen, and J. Kalbfleisch (2001). A modified likelihood ratio test for homogeneity in finite mixture models. *Journal of the Royal Statistical Society, Series B-Statistical Methodology 63*, 19–29.

Chen, H., J. Chen, and J. Kalbfleisch (2004). Testing for a finite mixture model with two components. *Journal of the Royal Statistical Society, Series B-Statistical Methodology 66*, 95–115.

Chen, J. (1998). Penalized likelihood-ratio test for finite mixture models with multinomial observations. *Can. J. Stat. 26*(4), 583–599.

Chen, J. and J. Kalbfleisch (2005). Modified likelihood ratio test in finite mixture models with a structural parameter. *Journal of statistical Planning and Inference 129*(1-2), 93–107.

Chung, K., T. Hughes, and L. Claxton (2000). Comparison of the mutagenic specificity induced by four nitro-group-containing aromatic amines in Salmonella typhimurium his genes. *Mutat Res 465*(1-2), 165–71.

Clayton, D. and J. Kaldor (1987). Empirical Bayes estimates for age-standardized relative risks. *Biometrics 43*, 671–681.

Cohen, J. (1988). *Statistical power analysis for the behavioral sciences.* (2nd ed.). Lawrence Earlbaum Associates. Hillsdale, NJ.

Cooley, J. and J. Tukey (1965). An algorithm for the machine calculation of complex Fourier series. *Mathematics of Computation 19*, 297–301.

Copas, J. and J. Shi (2001). A sensitivity analysis for publication bias in systematic review. *Med Res 10*, 251–65.

Cotterchio, M., N. Kreiger, M. Sloan, and A. Steingart (2001). Nonsteroidal anti-inflammatory drug use and breast cancer risk. *Cancer Epidemiol.Biomarkers Prev. 10*, 1213–1217.

Cox, D. and D. Hinkley (1974). *Theoretical statistics*. London: Chapman & Hall Ltd.

Davidian, M. and D. Giltinan (1995). *Nonlinear Models for Repeated Measurement Data*. London, UK: Chapman & Hall.

DeGeorge, B. and W. Koch (2007). Beta blocker specificity: a building block toward personalized medicine. *J Clin Invest 117*(1), 86–9.

Dempster, A., N. Laird, and D. Rubin (1977). Maximum likelihood from incomplete data via the EM algorithm. Discussion. *J. R. Stat. Soc., Ser. B 39*, 1–38.

Denkert, C., K. J. Winzer, and S. Hauptmann (2004). Prognostic impact of cyclooxygenase-2 in breast cancer. *Clin. Breast Cancer 4*, 428–433.

DerSimonian, R. (1986). Algorithm AS221: Maximum likelihood estimation of a mixing distribution. *J. R. Stat. Soc., Ser. C 35*, 302–309.

DerSimonian, R. and N. Laird (1986). Meta-analysis in clinical trials. *Controlled Clin Trials 7*, 177–188.

Der Spiegel (1996). *20*, 66–67.

Dias, J. and M. Wedel (2004). An empirical comparison of EM, SEM and MCMC performance for problematic Gaussian mixture likelihoods. *Statistics and Computing 14*(4), 323–332.

Dickersin, K. (2002). Systematic reviews in epidemiology: why are we so far behind? *International Journal of Epidemiology 31*, 6–12.

Dickersin, K., R. Scherer, and C. Lefebvre (1994). Identifying relevant studies for systematic reviews. *BMJ 309*, 1286–1291.

Dieckmann, H. (1992). Incidence of leukemia in the Elbmarsch area. *Gesundheitswesen 54*(10), 592–6.

Diggle, P. J. (1990). *Time series. A biostatistical introduction*. Oxford Science Publications; Oxford Statistical Science Series, 5. Oxford: Clarendon Press. xi, 257 p.

Dobson, A. (2008). *An introduction to generalized linear models* (Third ed.). London etc.: Chapman & Hall. x, 174 p.

Dorgan, J., N. Boakye, T. Fears, R. Schleicher, W. Helsel, C. Anderson, J. Robinson, J. Guin, S. Lessin, L. Ratnasinghe, and J. Tangrea (2004). Serum carotenoids and alpha-tocopherol and risk of nonmelanoma skin cancer. *Cancer Epidemiol Biomarkers Prev 13*(8), 1276–82.

Dumouchel, W. (1995). Meta-analysis for dose-response models. *Stat Med 14*(5-7), 679–85.

Eckardt, F. and R. Haynes (1977). Kinetics of mutation induction by ultraviolet light in excision-deficient yeast. *Genetics 85*(2), 225–47.

Efron, B. (1979). Bootstrap methods: Another look at the jackknife. *Ann. Stat. 7*, 1–26.

Efron, B. (1982). *The jackknife, the bootstrap and other resampling plans*. CBMS-NSF Reg. Conf. Ser. Appl. Math. 38.

Efron, B. (2004). Large Scale Simultaneous Hypothesis Testing: The Choice of a Null Hypothesis. *Journal of the American Statistical Association 99*(465), 96–104.

Efron, B. and R. Tibshirani (1986). Bootstrap methods for standard errors, confidence intervals, and other measures of statistical accuracy. *Stat. Sci. 1*, 54–77.

Efron, B. and R. Tibshirani (2002). Empirical bayes methods and false discovery rates for microarrays. *Genet Epidemiol 23*(1), 70–86.

Efron, B., R. Tibshirani, J. D. Storey, and V. Tusher (2001). Empirical Bayes Analysis of Microarray Experiment. *Journal of the American Statistical Association 96*(456), 1151–1160.

Efron, B. and R. J. Tibshirani (1993). *An introduction to the bootstrap*. Monographs on Statistics and Applied Probability. 57. New York, NY: Chapman & Hall.

Egger, M., G. Davey-Smith, and D. Altman (2001). *Systematic Reviews in Health Care. Meta-analysis in context. 2nd ed.* BMJ Publishing Group.

Egger, M., G. Davey-Smith, and M. Schneider (2001). *Systematic reviews of observational studies*, pp. 211–227. London, BMJ Publishing Group.

Egger, M., G. Davey Smith, M. Schneider, and C. Minder (1997). Bias in meta-analysis detected by a simple, graphical test. *BMJ 315*(7109), 629–34.

Egger, M., M. Schneider, and G. Smith (1998). Spurious precision? Meta-analysis of observational studies. *BMJ 316*, 140–144.

Eilers, P. (1995). Indirect observations, composite link models and penalized likelihood. In G. Seeber, B. Francis, R. Hatzinger, and G. Steckel-Berger (Eds.), *Statistical Modelling*, pp. 91–98. Springer, Berlin.

Elliott, P., J. Wakefield, N. Best, and D. Briggs (Eds.) (2000). *Spatial Epidemiology - Methods and Applications*. Oxford University Press, Oxford.

Everitt, B. (1984). Maximum likelihood estimation of the parameters in the mixture of two univariate normal distributions: a comparison of different algorithms. *The Statistician 33*, 205–215.

Everitt, B. and D. Hand (1981). *Finite Mixture Distributions*. Monographs on Applied Probability and Statistics. London, New York: Chapman and Hall.

Faure, H., P. Preziosi, A. Roussel, S. Bertrais, P. Galan, S. Hercberg, and A. Favier (2006). Factors influencing blood concentration of retinol, alpha-tocopherol, vitamin C, and beta-carotene in the French participants of the SU.VI.MAX trial. *Eur J Clin Nutr 60*(6), 706–17.

Fawzi, W. W., T. C. Chalmers, M. G. Herrera, and F. Mosteller (1993). Vitamin A supplementation and child mortality. A meta-analysis. *JAMA 269*(7), 898–903.

Feinstein, A. (1995). Meta-analysis: statistical alchemy for the 21st century. *J Clin Epidemiol 48*, 71–79.

Feller, W. (1968). *An Introduction to Probability Theory and its Applications, Vol. I*. Wiley, New York.

Feng, Z. and C. McCulloch (1996). Using bootstrap likelihood ratios in finite mixture models. *J. R. Stat. Soc., Ser. B 58*(3), 609–617.

Feng, Z. and C. E. McCulloch (1992). Statistical inference using maximum likelihood estimation and the generalized likelihood ratio when the true parameter is on the boundary of the parameter space. *Stat. Probab. Lett. 13*(4), 325–332.

Feng, Z. and C. E. McCulloch (1994). On the likelihood ratio test statistic for the number of components in a normal mixture with unequal variances. *Biometrics 50*(4), 1158–1162.

Flusser, D., E. Zylber-Katz, L. Granit, and M. Levy (1988). Influence of food on the pharmacokinetics of dipyrone. *European Journal of Clinical Pharmacology 34*, 105–107.

Frühwirth-Schnatter, S. (2006). *Finite mixture and Markov switching models*. Springer Series in Statistics. Berlin: Springer. xix, 492 p.

Fu, Y. J., J. H. Chen, and J. D. Kalbfleisch (2006). Testing for homogeneity in genetic linkage analysis. *Statistica Sinica 16*(3), 805–823.

Garcia Rodriguez, L. A. and A. Gonzalez-Perez (2004). Risk of breast cancer among users of aspirin and other anti-inflammatory drugs. *Br. J. Cancer 91*, 525–529.

Gardner, M., M. Snee, A. Hall, C. Powell, S. Downes, and J. Terrell (1990). Results of case-control study of leukaemia and lymphoma among young people near Sellafield nuclear plant in West Cumbria. *BMJ 300*(6722), 423–9.

Garel, B. (2007). Recent asymptotic results in testing for mixtures. *Computational Statisics & Data Analysis 51*(11), 5295–5304.

Gasser, T. and L. Molinari (1996). The analysis of the EEG. *Stat Methods Med Res. 5*, 67–99.

Gentleman, R., V. Carey, W. Huber, R. Irizarry, and S. Dudoit (Eds.) (2005). *Bioinformatics and Computational Biology Solutions Using R and Bioconductor*. Springer, Berlin.

Gibaldi, M. and D. Perrier (1982). *Pharmacokinetics* (second ed.). New York, NY: Marcel Dekker.

Glass, G. (1976). Primary, Secondary and Meta-Analysis of research. *Educational Researcher 5*, 3–8.

Glass, G. (1977). Integrating findings: The meta-analysis of research. *Rev Res 5*, 3–8.

Goffinet, B., P. Loisel, and B. Laurent (1992). Testing in normal mixture models when the proportions are known. *Biometrika 79*(4), 842–846.

Golub, T., D. Slonim, P. Tamayo, C. Huard, M. Gaasenbeek, J. Mesirov, H. Coller, M. Loh, J. Downing, M. Caligiuri, C. Bloomfield, and E. Lander (1999). Molecular classification of cancer: class discovery and class prediction by gene expression monitoring. *Science 286*(5439), 531–7.

Gonzalez-Perez, A., L. A. Garcia Rodriguez, and R. Lopez-Ridaura (2003). Effects of non-steroidal anti-inflammatory drugs on cancer sites other than the colon and rectum: a meta-analysis. *BMC. Cancer 3*, 28.

Goodman, G., G. Omenn, M. Thornquist, B. Lund, B. Metch, and I. Gylys-Colwell (1993). The Carotene and Retinol Efficacy Trial (CARET) to prevent lung cancer in high-risk populations: pilot study with cigarette smokers. *Cancer Epidemiol Biomarkers Prev 2*(4), 389–96.

Goodman, G., M. Thornquist, J. Balmes, M. Cullen, F. Meyskens, Jr, G. Omenn, B. Valanis, and J. Williams, Jr (2004). The Beta-Carotene and Retinol Efficacy Trial: incidence of lung cancer and cardiovascular disease mortality during 6-year follow-up after stopping beta-carotene and retinol supplements. *J Natl Cancer Inst 96*(23), 1743–50.

Goodman, G., M. Thornquist, M. Kestin, B. Metch, G. Anderson, and G. Omenn (1996). The association between participant characteristics and serum concentrations of beta-carotene, retinol, retinyl palmitate, and alpha-tocopherol among participants in the Carotene and Retinol Efficacy Trial (CARET) for prevention of lung cancer. *Cancer Epidemiol Biomarkers Prev 5*(10), 815–21.

Gottardo, R., A. Raftery, K. Yeung, and R. Bumgarner (2006). Bayesian robust inference for differential gene expression in microarrays with multiple samples. *Biometrics 62*(1), 10–8.

Greaves, M. F. (1988). Speculations on the cause of childhood acute lymphoblastic leukemia. *Leukemia 2*(2), 120–5.

Greaves, M. F. (1997). Aetiology of acute leukaemia. *Lancet 349*(9048), 344–9.

Greaves, M. F. and F. E. Alexander (1993). An infectious etiology for common acute lymphoblastic leukemia in childhood? *Leukemia 7*(3), 349–60.

Greenland, S. (1987). Quantitative methods in the review of epidemiologic literature. *Epidemiol Rev 9*, 1–302.

Greenland, S. (1994). Invited commentary: a critical look at some popular meta-analytic methods. *Am J Epidemiol 140*, 290–296.

Greenland, S. and M. P. Longnecker (1992). Methods for trend estimation from summarized dose-response data, with applications to meta-analysis. *Am. J. Epidemiol. 135*, 1301–1309.

Hamza, T. H., H. C. van Houwelingen, and T. Stijnen (2008). The binomial distribution of meta-analysis was preferred to model within-study variability. *J Clin Epidemiol 61*(1), 41–51.

Hardy, R. and S. Thompson (1996). A likelihood approach to meta-analysis with random effects. *Stat Med 15*(6), 619–29.

Harris, R. E., G. A. Alshafie, H. Abou-Issa, and K. Seibert (2000). Chemoprevention of breast cancer in rats by celecoxib, a cyclooxygenase 2 inhibitor. *Cancer Res. 60*, 2101–2103.

Harris, R. E., J. Beebe-Donk, H. Doss, and D. D. Burr (2005). Aspirin, ibuprofen, and other non-steroidal anti-inflammatory drugs in cancer prevention: a critical review of non-selective cox-2 blockade (review). *Oncol. Rep. 13*, 559–583.

Harris, R. E., R. T. Chlebowski, R. D. Jackson, D. J. Frid, J. L. Ascenseo, G. Anderson, A. Loar, R. J. Rodabough, E. White, and A. McTiernan (2003). Breast cancer and nonsteroidal anti-inflammatory drugs: prospective results from the women's health initiative. *Cancer Res. 63*, 6096–6101.

Hedenmalm, K. and O. Spigset (2002). Agranulocytosis and other blood dyscrasias associated with dipyrone (metamizole). *European Journal of Clinical Pharmacology 58*, 265–274.

Herrmann, W. M., K. Fichte, and S. Kubicki (1978). [The mathematical rationale for the clinical EEG-frequency-bands. 1. Factor analysis with EEG-power estimations for determining frequency bands]. *EEG EMG Z Elektroenzephalogr Elektromyogr Verwandte Geb 9*(3), 146–54.

Hill, A. (1965). The environment and disease: association or causation? *Proceedings of the Royal Society of Medicine 58*, 295–300.

Hill, H. and D. Kleinbaum (2000). *Bias in observational studies*, pp. 94–100. John Wiley and Sons, Chichester.

Hills, M. and F. Alexander (1989). Statistical methods used in assessing the risk of disease near a point source of possible environmental pollution: a review. *Journal of the Royal Statistical Society, Series A 152*, 353–363.

Hiriart-Urruty, JB. and Lemarichal, C (2001). *Fundamentals of Convex Analysis*. Springer, Berlin.

Hoffmann, W., H. Dieckmann, and I. Schmitz-Feuerhake (1997). A cluster of childhood leukemia near a nuclear reactor in northern Germany. *Arch Environ Health 52*(4), 275–80.

Hoffmann, W. and P. Schlattmann (1999). An analysis of the geographical distribution of leukaemia incidence in the vicinity of a suspected point source: a case study. In A. Lawson, A. Biggeri, D. Böhning, E. Lesaffre, J. F. Viel, and R. Bertollini (Eds.), *Disease Mapping and Risk Assessment for Public Health decision making*, pp. 395–410. Wiley, Chichester.

Holland, W. (Ed.) (1993). *European Community Atlas of Avoidable Death, Vol. 2*. Oxford Universit Press, Oxford.

Hothorn, L. and F. Bretz (2003). Dose-response and thresholds in mutagenicity studies: a statistical testing approach. *Altern Lab Anim 31 Suppl 1*, 97–103.

Huber, P. (1967). The Behaviour of Maximum Likelihood Estimates under Nonstandard Conditions. In *Proceedings of the 5th Berkeley symposium*, Number 1, pp. 221–233.

Huedo-Medina, T., J. Sanchez-Meca, F. Marin-Martinez, and J. Botella (2006). Assessing heterogeneity in meta-analysis: Q statistic or I2 index? *Psychol Methods 11*(2), 193–206.

Hung, R., P. Boffetta, and J. Brockmoller (2003). CYP1A1 and GSTM1 genetic polymorphisms and lung cancer risk in caucasian non-smokers: a pooled analysis. *Carcinogenesis 24*, 875–82.

IAAAS (1986). Risks of agranulocytosis and aplastic anemia. A first report of their relation to drug use with special reference to analgesics. The International Agranulocytosis and Aplastic Anemia Study. *JAMA 256*(13), 1749–1757.

Iganaki, N. (1973). Asymptotic relations between the likelihood estimating function and the maximum likelihood estimator. *Ann. Inst. Stat. Math. 265*, 1–26.

Il'yasova, D., I. Hertz-Picciotto, U. Peters, J. A. Berlin, and C. Poole (2005). Choice of exposure scores for categorical regression in meta-analysis: a case study of a common problem. *Cancer Causes Control 16*, 383–388.

Jackson, D. (2006). The power of the standard test for the presence of heterogeneity in meta-analysis. *Stat Med 25*(15), 2688–99.

Jamshidian, M. and R. I. Jennrich (1993). Conjugate gradient acceleration of the EM algorithm. *J. Am. Stat. Assoc. 88*(421), 221–228.

Jamshidian, M. and R. I. Jennrich (1997). Acceleration of the EM algorithm by using quasi-Newton methods. *J. R. Stat. Soc., Ser. B 59*(3), 569–587.

Jewell, N. P. (1982). Mixtures of exponential distributions. *Ann. Stat. 10*, 479–484.

Jiang, D. and N. Zhao (2006). A clinical prognostic prediction of lymph node-negative breast cancer by gene expression profiles. *J Cancer Res Clin Oncol 132*(9), 579–87.

Joe, H. and R. Zhu (2005). Generalized Poisson distribution: the property of mixture of Poisson and comparison with negative binomial distribution. *Biom J 47*(2), 219–29.

Johnson, N. L., S. Kotz, and A. W. Kemp (1992). *Univariate discrete distributions. 2. ed*. Wiley Series in Probability and Mathematical Statistics. Probability and Mathematical Statistics. New York: John Wiley & Sons. 565 p.

Johnson, T. W., K. E. Anderson, D. Lazovich, and A. R. Folsom (2002). Association of aspirin and nonsteroidal anti-inflammatory drug use with breast cancer. *Cancer Epidemiol.Biomarkers Prev. 11*, 1586–1591.

Jones, M. P., T. W. O'Gorman, J. H. Lemke, and R. F. Woolson (1989). A Monte Carlo investigation of homogeneity tests of the odds ratio under various sample size configurations. *Biometrics 45*(1), 171–81.

Jones, P. N. and G. J. McLachlan (1990). Maximum likelihood estimation from grouped and truncated data with finite normal mixture models. *J. R. Stat. Soc., Ser. C 39*(2), 273–282.

Kaatsch, P., U. Kaletsch, R. Meinert, and J. Michaelis (1998). An extended study on childhood malignancies in the vicinity of german nuclear power plants. *Cancer Causes Control. 9*, 529–533.

Kaatsch, P., C. Spix, R. Schulze-Rath, S. Schmiedel, and M. Blettner (2008). Leukaemia in young children living in the vicinity of German nuclear power plants. *Int J Cancer 22*, 721–726.

Karlis, D. and E. Xekalaki (1999). On testing for the number of components in a mixed Poisson model. *Ann. Inst. Stat. Math. 51*(1), 149–162.

Karlis, D. and E. Xekalaki (2003). Choosing initial values for the EM algorithm for finite mixtures. *Computational Statistics and Data Analysis 41*(3-4), 577–590.

Khuder, S. A. and A. B. Mutgi (2001). Breast cancer and NSAID use: a meta-analysis. *Br. J. Cancer 84*, 1188–1192.

Kiefer, J. and J. Wolfowitz (1956). Consistency of the maximum likelihood estimator in the presence of infinitely many incidental parameters. *Ann. Math. Statistics 27*, 887–906.

Kim, B. and B. Margolin (1999). Statistical methods for the Ames Salmonella assay: a review. *Mutat Res 436*(1), 113–22.

Kinlen, L. (1988). Evidence for an infective cause of childhood leukaemia: comparison of a Scottish new town with nuclear reprocessing sites in Britain. *Lancet 2*(8624), 1323–7.

Kinlen, L. (1997). Infection and childhood leukaemia near nuclear sites. *Lancet 349*(9066), 1702.

Kirkpatrick, S., C. D. Gelatt, and M. P. Vecchi (1983). Optimization by simulated annealing. *Science 220*(4598), 671–680.

Knapp, G., B. Biggerstaff, and J. Hartung (2006). Assessing the amount of heterogeneity in random-effects meta-analysis. *Biom J 48*(2), 271–85.

Knapp, G. and J. Hartung (2003). Improved tests for a random effects meta-regression with a single covariate. *Stat Med 22*(17), 2693–710.

Krewski, D., B. Leroux, S. Bleuer, and L. Broekhoven (1993). Modeling the Ames Salmonella/microsome assay. *Biometrics 49*(2), 499–510.

Kroemer, H., G. Mikus, and M. Eichelbaum (1994). Clinical relevance of pharmacogenetics. In P. G. Welling and L. P. Balant (Eds.), *Pharmacokinetics of Drugs*, Chapter 9. Berlin, Germany: Springer-Verlag.

Lagiou, P., V. Benetou, N. Tebelis, A. Papas, A. Naska, and A. Trichopoulou (2003). Plasma carotenoid levels in relation to tobacco smoking and demographic factors. *Int J Vitam Nutr Res 73*(3), 226–31.

Lai, T. L. and M. C. Shih (2003). Nonparametric estimation in nonlinear mixed effects models. *Biometrika 90*(1), 1–13.

Laird, N. M. (1978). Nonparametric maximum likelihood estimation of a mixing distribution. *J. Am. Stat. Assoc. 73*, 805–811.

Lange, K. (1995). A quasi-Newton acceleration of the EM algorithm. *Stat. Sin. 5*(1), 1–18.

Lange, K. (2004). *Optimization*. Springer Texts in Statistics. New York, NY: Springer. xiii, 252 p.

Last, J. (Ed.) (2000). *A Dictionary of Epidemiology*. Oxford University Press.

Lawless, J. (1987). Negative binomial and mixed poisson regression. *Canadian Journal of Statistics-Revue Canadienne de statistique 15*(3), 209–225.

Lawson, A. B. (1993). On the analysis of mortality events associated with a prespecified fixed point. *J R Stat Soc, Ser A Stat Soc. 156*, 363–377.

Lawson, A. B., A. Biggeri, D. Boehning, E. Lesaffre, J. Viel, A. Clark, P. Schlattmann, and F. Divino (2000). Disease mapping models: an empirical evaluation. Disease Mapping Collaborative Group. *Stat Med 19*(17-18), 2217–41.

Lawson, A. B., A. Biggeri, D. Böhning, E. Lesaffre, J. F. Viel, and R. Bertollini (Eds.) (1999). *Disease Mapping and Risk Assessment for Public Health Decision Making*. Wiley, Chichester.

Lawson, A. B., F. L. Williams, and Y. Liu (2007). Some simple tests for spatial effects around putative sources of health risk. *Biom J 49*(4), 493–504.

Lawson, A. B. (2006). *Statistical Methods in Spatial Epidemiology*. Wiley, Chichester.

L'Ecuyer, P. (1988). Efficient and portable combined random number generators. *C.A.C.M. 31*, 742–749.

Lee, M. L., F. C. Kuo, G. A. Whitmore, and J. Sklar (2000). Importance of replication in microarray gene expression studies: statistical methods and evidence from repetitive cDNA hybridizations. *Proc Natl Acad Sci U S A 97*(18), 9834–9.

Leroux, B. G. and M. L. Puterman (1992). Maximum-Penalized-Likelihood Estimation for Independent and Markov-Dependent Mixture models. *Biometrics 48*, 545–558.

Levy, M., M. Muszkat, B. Rich, B. Rosenkranz, and P. Schlattmann (2007). Population Pharmacokinetic Analysis of the active metabolite of Dipyrone. *submitted*.

Levy, M., E. Zylber-Katz, and B. Rosenkranz (1995). Clinical pharmacokinetics of dipyrone and its metabolites. *Clin. Pharmacokin. 28*(3), 216–234.

Leyland, A. and C. Davies (2005). Empirical Bayes methods for disease mapping. *Statistical Methods in Medical Research 14*(1), 17–34.

Liang, K.-Y. and S. Zeger (1986). Longitudinal Data Analysis Using Generalized Linear Models. *Biometrika 73*, 13–22.

Lindsay, B. G. (1983a). The geometry of mixture likelihoods: A general theory. *Ann. Stat. 11*, 86–94.

Lindsay, B. G. (1983b). The geometry of mixture likelihoods, part ii: The exponential family. *Ann. Stat. 11*, 783–792.

Lindsay, B. G. (1995). *Mixture models Theory, Geometry and Applications*. NSF-CBMS regional conference series in probability and statistics, vol. 5. Hayward: Institute of Statistical Mathematics.

Lindsay, B. G. and M. L. Lesperance (1995). A review of semiparametric mixture models. *J. Stat. Plann. Inference 47*(1-2), 29–39.

Lindsay, B. G. and K. Roeder (1992). Residual diagnostics for mixture models. *J. Am. Stat. Assoc. 87*(419), 785–794.

Liu, C. and D. B. Rubin (1994). The ECME algorithm: A simple extension of EM and ECM with faster monotone convergence. *Biometrika 81*(4), 633–648.

Lo, K. and R. Gottardo (2007). Flexible empirical Bayes models for differential gene expression. *Bioinformatics 23*(3), 328–35.

Lo, Y. (2005). Likelihood ratio tests of the number of components in a normal mixture with unequal variances. *Statistics and Probabiliity Letters 71*(3), 225–235.

Lo, Y., N. R. Mendell, and D. B. Rubin (2001). Testing the number of components in a normal mixture. *Biometrika 88*(3), 767–778.

Louis, T. A. (1982). Finding the observed information matrix when using the EM algorithm. *J. R. Stat. Soc., Ser. B 44*, 226–233.

Lubin, J., J. Boice, JD, C. Edling, R. Hornung, G. Howe, E. Kunz, R. Kusiak, H. Morrison, E. Radford, J. Samet, and et al. (1995). Radon-exposed underground miners and inverse dose-rate (protraction enhancement) effects. *Health Phys 69*, 494–500.

Lumley, T. (2008). *rmeta: Meta-analysis*. R package version 2.14.

Lunn, D., N. Best, A. Thomas, J. Wakefield, and D. Spiegelhalter (2002). Bayesian analysis of population PK/PD models: general concepts and software. *J Pharmacokinet Pharmacodyn 29*(3), 271–307.

Lunn, D. J., J. Wakefield, A. Thomas, N. Best, and S. David (1999). PKBugs user guide (version 1.1).

Macaskill, P., S. Walter, and L. Irwig (2001). A comparison of methods to detect publication bias in meta-analysis. *Statistics in Medicine 20*, 641–654.

Mallet, A. (1986). A maximum likelihood estimation method for random coefficient regression models. *Biometrika 73*, 645–656.

Mangiapane, S., M. Blettner, and P. Schlattmann (2008). Aspirin use and breast cancer risk: a meta-analysis and meta-regression of observational studies from 2001 to 2005. *Pharmacoepidemiol Drug Saf 17*(2), 115–24.

Margetts, B. and A. Jackson (1996). The determinants of plasma beta-carotene: interaction between smoking and other lifestyle factors. *Eur J Clin Nutr 50*(4), 236–8.

Margolin, B., N. Kaplan, and E. Zeiger (1981). Statistical analysis of the Ames Salmonella/microsome test. *Proc Natl Acad Sci U S A 78*(6), 3779–83.

Margolin, B. H., B. S. Kim, and K. J. Risko (1989). The Ames Salmonella Microsome Mutagenicity Assay: Issues of Inference and Validation. *Journal of the American Statistical Association 84*, 651–661.

Marshall, S. F., L. Bernstein, H. Anton-Culver, D. Deapen, P. L. Horn-Ross, H. Mohrenweiser, D. Peel, R. Pinder, D. M. Purdie, P. Reynolds, D. Stram, D. West, W. E. Wright, A. Ziogas, and R. K. Ross (2005, Jun). Nonsteroidal anti-inflammatory drug use and breast cancer risk by stage and hormone receptor status. *J.Natl.Cancer Inst. 97*, 805–812.

Martuzzi, M. and M. Hills (1995). Estimating the degree of heterogeneity between event rates using likelihood. *Am J Epidemiol 141*(4), 369–74.

Maylath, E., J. Seidel, and P. Schlattmann (2000a). Inequity in the hospital care of patients with alcoholism and medication addiction. *Eur Addict Res 6*(2), 79–83.

Maylath, E., J. Seidel, and P. Schlattmann (2000b). Spatial distribution of in-patient service use of psychiatric patients: somatic departments versus psychiatric units. *Soc Psychiatry Psychiatr Epidemiol 35*(9), 408–17.

McCormick, D. L., M. J. Madigan, and R. C. Moon (1985, Apr). Modulation of rat mammary carcinogenesis by indomethacin. *Cancer Res. 45*, 1803–1808.

McCullagh, P. and J. Nelder (1989). *Generalized linear models. 2nd ed.* Monographs on Statistics and Applied Probability. 37. London etc.: Chapman and Hall. xix, 511 p.

McCulloch, C. E. and S. R. Searle (2001). *Generalized, Linear, and Mixed Models.* Wiley.

McLachlan, G. J. and N. Khan (2004). On a resampling approach for tests on the number of clusters with mixture model-based clustering of tissue samples. *Journal of multivariate analysis 90*(1), 90–105.

McLachlan, G. J., C. McLaren, and D. Matthews (1995). An algorithm for the likelihood ratio test of one versus two components in a normal mixture model fitted to grouped und truncated data. *Commun. Stat., Simulation Comput. 24*(4), 965–985.

McLachlan, G. J. and D. Peel (2000). *Finite Mixture Models.* Wiley Series in Probability and Mathematical Statistics. Applied Probability and Statistics. Chichester: Wiley. xxii, 419 p.

McLachlan, G. J. and K. E. Basford (1988). *Mixture models: Inference and Applications to Clustering.* Statistics: Textbooks and Monographs, 84. New York etc.: Marcel Dekker, Inc. xi, 253 p.

McLachlan, G. J., R. W. Bean, and L. B. Jones (2006). A simple implementation of a normal mixture approach to differential gene expression in multiclass microarrays. *Bioinformatics 22*(13), 1608–15.

McLachlan, G. J., K.-A. Do, and C. Ambroise (2004). *Analyzing Microarray Gene Expression Data.* Wiley, Chichester.

McLachlan, G. J. and T. Krishnan (1997). *The EM algorithm and Extensions.* Wiley Series in Probability and Mathematical Statistics. Applied Probability and Statistics.

Meilijson, I. (1989). A fast improvement to the EM algorithm on its own terms. *J. R. Stat. Soc., Ser. B 51*(1), 127–138.

Mendell, N. R., H. C. Thode, and S. J. Finch (1991). The likelihood ratio test for the two-component normal mixture problem: power and sample size analysis. *Biometrics 47*, 1143–1148.

Meng, X.-L. and D. B. Rubin (1993). Maximum likelihood estimation via the ECM algorithm: A general framework. *Biometrika 80*(2), 267–278.

Meng, X.-L. and D. van Dyk (1997). The EM algorithm - an old folk-song sung to a fast new tune. *J. R. Stat. Soc., Ser. B 59*(3), 511–567.

Metropolis, N., A. Rosenbluth, M. Rosenbluth, A. Teller, and E. Teller (1953). The Monte Carlo method. *Journal of the American Statistical Association* (44), 335–341.

Michaelis, J. (1998). Recent epidemiological studies on ionizing radiation and childhood cancer in Germany. *Int J Radiat Biol 73*(4), 377–81.

Michaelis, J., B. Keller, G. Haaf, and P. Kaatsch (1992). Incidence of childhood malignancies in the vicinity of west german nuclear power plants. *Cancer Causes Control 3*, 255–263.

Möhner, M. R., Stabenow, and B. Eisinger (1994). *Atlas der Krebsinzidenz in der DDR 1961-1989.* Ullstein-Mosby, Berlin.

Mollie, A. and S. Richardson (1991). Empirical Bayes estimates of cancer mortality rates using spatial models. *Stat Med 10*(1), 95–112.

Mood, A. M., F. A. Graybill, and D. C. Boes (1974). *Introduction to the theory of statistics. 3rd ed.* McGraw-Hill Series in Probability and Statistics. New York etc.: McGraw- Hill Book Company. XVI, 564 p. $ 12.50.

Moran, P. (1948). The interpretation of statistical maps. *Journal of the Royal Statistical Society, Series B 10*, 243–251.

Mortelmans, K. and E. Zeiger (2000). The Ames Salmonella/microsome mutagenicity assay. *Mutat Res 455*(1-2), 29–60.

Muirhead, C. (2006). Methods for detecting disease clustering, with consideration of childhood leukaemia. *Stat Methods Med Res 15*(4), 363–83.

Nelder, J. and R. Wedderburn (1972). Generalized linear models. *Journal of the Royal Statistical Society, Series A 135*, 370–84.

Newton, M., C. Kendziorski, C. Richmond, F. Blattner, and K. Tsui (2001). On differential variability of expression ratios: improving statistical inference about gene expression changes from microarray data. *J Comput Biol 8*(1), 37–52.

Newton, M. A., A. Noueiry, D. Sarkar, and P. Ahlquist (2004). Detecting differential gene expression with a semiparametric hierarchical mixture method. *Biostatistics 5*(2), 155–76.

Ng, S. and G. J. McLachlan (2003). An EM-based semi-parametric mixture model approach to the regression analysis of competing-risks data. *Stat Med 22*(7), 1097–111.

Ng, S. and G. J. McLachlan (2004). Speeding up the EM algorithm for mixture model-based segmentation of magnetic resonance images. *Pattern Recognition 37*(8), 1573–1589.

Nierenberg, D., T. Stukel, J. Baron, B. Dain, and E. Greenberg (1989). Determinants of plasma levels of beta-carotene and retinol. Skin Cancer Prevention Study Group. *Am J Epidemiol 130*(3), 511–21.

Nityasuddhi, D. and D. Böhning (2003). Asymptotic properties of the EM algorithm estimate for normal mixture models with component specific variances. *Computational Statistics & Data Analysis 41*(3-4), 591–601.

Normand, S. (1999). Meta-analysis: formulating, evaluating, combining, and reporting. *Stat Med 18*, 321–59.

Notari, R. E. (1975). *Biopharmaceutics and Pharmacokinetics: An Introduction* (second ed.). New York, NY: Marcel Dekker.

Olkin, I. (1994). Invited commentary: Re: "A critical look at some popular meta-analytic methods". *Am J Epidemiol 140*, 297–299.

Parkin, D. M., F. Bray, J. Ferlay, and P. Pisani (2005, Mar). Global cancer statistics, 2002. *CA Cancer J.Clin. 55*, 74–108.

Parmigiani, G and Garett ES and Irizarry, R. (Ed.) (2003). *The Analysis of Gene Expression Data - Methods and Software*. Springer.

Paul, S. and A. Donner (1989). A comparison of tests of homogeneity of odds ratios in k 2x2 tables. *Stat Med 8*, 1455–1468.

Pelkonen, O. and D. Breimer (1994). Role of environmental factors in the pharmacokinetics of drugs: Considerations with respect to animal models, p-450 enzymes, and probe drugs. In P. G. Welling and L. P. Balant (Eds.), *Pharmacokinetics of Drugs*, Chapter 10, pp. 289–332. Berlin, Germany: Springer-Verlag.

Peters, J., A. Sutton, D. Jones, K. Abrams, and L. Rushton (2006). Comparison of two methods to detect publication bias in meta-analysis. *JAMA 295*(6), 676–80.

Pettiti, D. (1994). *Meta-Analysis, Decision Analysis and Cost-Effectiveness Analysis*. Oxford University Press.

Pilla, R. S. and B. G. Lindsay (2001). Alternative *EM* methods for nonparametric finite mixture models. *Biometrika 88*(2), 535–550.

Pinheiro, J. and D. Bates (1995). Approximations to the log-likelihood function in the nonlinear mixed effects model. *Journal of Computational and Graphical Statistics 4*, 12–35.

Pinheiro, J. and D. Bates (2000). *Mixed-effects models in S and S-Plus*. Statistics and Computing. New York, NY: Springer. xvi, 528 p.

Platt, R., B. Leroux, and N. Breslow (1999). Generalized linear mixed models for meta-analysis. *Stat Med 18*(6), 643–54.

Polymenis, A. and D. M. Titterington (1998). On the determination of the number of components in a mixture. *Stat. Probab. Lett. 38*(4), 295–298.

Potthoff, R. and M. Whittinghill (1966). Testing for homogeneity II. The Poisson distribution. *Biometrika 53*, 183–190.

Press, W. H., S. A. Teukolsky, W. T. Vetterling, and B. P. Flannery (2007). *Numerical recipes. The art of scientific computing* (Third ed.). Cambridge: Univ. Press.

Priestley, M. (1991). *Spectral analysis and time series. Volume 1: Univariate series. Volume 2: Multivariate series, prediction and control. Reprinted with corrections.* Probability and Mathematical Statistics. London etc.: Academic Press Inc., Harcourt Brace Jovanovich. xviii, 890 p., xli p.

Proust, C. and H. Jacqmin-Gadda (2005). Estimation of linear mixed models with a mixture of distribution for the random effects. *Comput Methods Programs Biomed 78*(2), 165–73.

Quinn, B., G. McLachlan, and N. Hjort (1987). A note on the Aitkin-Rubin approach to hypothesis testing in mixture models. *J. R. Stat. Soc., Ser. B 49*, 311–314.

R Development Core Team (2008). *R: A Language and Environment for Statistical Computing.* Vienna, Austria: R Foundation for Statistical Computing. ISBN 3-900051-07-0.

Rao, C. (1948). Large sample tests of statistical hypotheses concerning several parameters with applications to problems of estimation. *Proceeding of the Cambridge Philosophical Society 44*, 50–57.

Redner, R. and H. F. Walker (1984). Mixture densities, maximum likelihood and the EM-algorithm. *SIAM Review 20*, 195–239.

Richardson, S. and P. J. Green (1997). On Bayesian analysis of mixtures with an unknown number of components. (With discussion). *J. R. Stat. Soc., Ser. B 59*(4), 731–792.

Ridolfi, A. and J. Idier (1999). Penalized maximum likelihood estimation for univariate normal mixture distributions.

Riley, R., P. Lambert, J. Staessen, J. Wang, F. Gueyffier, L. Thijs, and F. Boutitie (2007). Meta-analysis of continuous outcomes combining individual patient data and aggregate data. *Stat Med.*

Robert, C. P. (1996). Mixtures of distributions: Inference and estimation. In Gilks, W. R. and Richardson, S. and Spiegelhalter, D. (Ed.), *Markov chain Monte Carlo in practice.*, pp. 441–464. Chapman and Hall, London.

Robert, P. and G. Casella (2004). *Monte Carlo Statistical Methods* (Second ed.). Springer, Berlin.

Rockafellar, R. (1993). Lagrange multipliers and optimality. *SIAM Rev. 35*(2), 183–238.

Rockafellar, R. (1996). *Convex Analysis.* Princeton University Press.

Roeder, K. (1994). A graphical technique for determining the number of components in a mixture of normals. *J. Am. Stat. Assoc. 89*(426), 487–495.

Rossouw, J., G. Anderson, R. Prentice, A. LaCroix, C. Kooperberg, M. Stefanick, R. Jackson, S. Beresford, B. Howard, K. Johnson, J. Kotchen, J. Ockene, and Writing Group for the Women's Health Initiative Investigators (2002). Risks and benefits of estrogen plus progestin in healthy postmenopausal women: principal results from the women's health initiative randomized controlled trial. *JAMA 288*, 321–33.

Rowland, M. and T. Tozer (2005). *Clinical Pharmacokinetics* (Third ed.). Lippincott, Williams and Wilkins.

Saha, K. and S. Paul (2005). Bias-corrected maximum likelihood estimator of the negative binomial dispersion parameter. *Biometrics 61*(1), 179–185.

Sauter, G. and R. Simon (2002). Predictive molecular pathology. *N Engl J Med 347*, 1995–1996.

Schelp, F., P. Vivatanasept, P. Sitaputra, S. Sornmani, P. Pongpaew, N. Vudhivai, S. Egormaiphol, and D. Bohning (1990). Relationship of the morbidity of under-fives to anthropometric measurements and community health intervention. *Trop Med Parasitol 41*(2), 121–126.

Schlattmann, P. (1996). The computer package DismapWin. *Statistics in Medicine 15*, 931.

Schlattmann, P. (2000). Mixture models and modelling heterogeneity of the regional distribution of avoidable death in Germany 1995. *Stud Health Technol Inform 77*, 417–22.

Schlattmann, P. (2003). Estimating the number of components in a finite mixture model: the special case of homogeneity. *Computational Statistics and Data Analysis 41*(3-4), 441–451.

Schlattmann, P. (2005). On bootstrapping the number of components in finite mixtures of Poisson distributions. *Statistics and Computing 15*(3), 179–188.

Schlattmann, P. and D. Bohning (1993). Computer packages C.A.MAN (Computer Assisted Mixture Analysis) and Dismap. *Statistics in Medicine 12*, 1965.

Schlattmann, P. and D. Böhning (1993). Mixture models and disease mapping. *Statistics in Medicine 12*, 943 –50.

Schlattmann, P. and D. Böhning (1997). On Bayesian analysis of mixtures with an unknown number of components. Contribution to a paper by S. Richardson and P.J. Green. *J. R. Stat. Soc., Ser. B 59*(4), 782–783.

Schlattmann, P., D. Böhning, A. Clark, and A. Lawson (1999). Lung cancer mortality in women in Germany 1995 - A case study in Disease Mapping. In A. Lawson, A. Biggeri, D. Böhning, E. Lesaffre, J. F. Viel, and R. Bertollini (Eds.), *Disease Mapping and Risk Assessment for Public Health decision making*. Wiley, Chichester.

Schlattmann, P., E. Dietz, and D. Böhning (1996). Covariate adjusted mixture models and disease mapping with the program DismapWin. *Statistics in Medicine 15*, 919–929.

Schlattmann, P., U. Malzahn, and D. Böhning (2003). META - A software package for meta-analysis in medicine, social sciences, and the pharmaceutical industry" in D. Böhning, K. H. Holling, and R. Schulze (Ed.). *"Meta-analysis: New developments and applications in medical and social sciences"*, Hogrefe und Huber Verlag, S. 251–258.

Schlittgen, R. and B. H. Streitberg (2001). *Zeitreihenanalyse. 9. unwesentlich veränderte Auflage, 9th. Ed* (9. ed.). München-Wien: R. Oldenbourg Verlag. XII, 505 S.

Schwarzer, G. (2007). *meta: Meta-Analysis*. R package version 0.8-2.

Schwarzer, G., G. Antes, and M. Schumacher (2002). Inflation of type I error rate in two statistical tests for the detection of publication bias in meta-analyses with binary outcomes. *Stat Med. 21*, 2465–77.

Seidel, W., K. Mosler, and M. Alker (2000a). A cautionary note on likelihood ratio tests in mixture models. *Ann. Inst. Stat. Math. 52*(3), 481–487.

Seidel, W., K. Mosler, and M. Alker (2000b). Likelihood ratio tests based on subglobal optimization: A power comparison in exponential mixture models. *Statistical Papers 41*(1), 85–98.

Seidel, W. and H. Sevcikova (2004). Types of likelihood maxima in mixture models and their implication on the performance of tests. *Annals of the Institute of Statistical Mathematics 56*(4), 631–654.

Seidel, W., K. Sever, and H. Sevcikova (2006). Efficient calculation of the NPMLE of a mixing distribution for mixtures of exponentials. *Computational Statistics and Data Analysis 50*, 1248–1271.

Senn, S. (2007). Trying to be precise about vagueness. *Stat Med 26*(7), 1417–30.

Shao, J. and D. Tu (1995). *The Jackknife and Bootstrap*. Springer Series in Statistics. New York, NY: Springer-Verlag.

Shapiro, S. (1994a). Is there is or is there ain't no baby?: Dr. Shapiro replies to Drs. Petitti and Greenland. *Am J Epidemiol 140*, 788–791.

Shapiro, S. (1994b). Meta-analysis/shmeta-analysis. *Am J Epidemiol 140*, 771–778.

Sheiner, L., H. Halkin, C. Peck, B. Rosenberg, and K. Melmon (1975). Improved computer-assisted digoxin therapy. A method using feedback of measured serum digoxin concentrations. *Ann Intern Med 82*(5), 619–27.

Sheiner, L., B. Rosenberg, and V. Marathe (1977). Estimation of population characteristics of pharmacokinetic parameters from routine clinical data. *J Pharmacokinet Biopharm 5*(5), 445–79.

Sheiner, L., B. Rosenberg, and K. Melmon (1972). Modelling of individual pharmacokinetics for computer-aided drug dosage. *Comput Biomed Res 5*(5), 411–59.

Sheiner, L. B. and T. H. Grasela, Jr. (1991). An introduction to mixed effect modeling: Concepts, definitions, and justifications. *Journal of Pharmacokinetics and Biopharmaceutics 19*(3, supplement).

Sidik, K. and J. Jonkman (2005). Simple heterogeneity estimation for meta-analysis. *Appl. Statist. 54*, 367–384.

Sidik, K. and J. Jonkman (2007). A comparison of heterogeneity variance estimators in combining results of studies. *Stat Med 26*(9), 1964–81.

Sillero-Arenas, M., M. Delgado-Rodriguez, R. Rodiguesw-Canteras, A. Bueno-Cavanillas, and R. Galvez-Vargas (1992). Menopausal hormone replacement therapy and breast cancer: a meta-analysis. *Obstet Gynecol. 79*, 286–294.

Silverman, B. W. (1981). Using kernel density estimates to investigate multimodality. *J. R. Stat. Soc., Ser. B 43*, 97–99.

Simar, L. (1976). Maximum likelihood estimation of a compound Poisson process. *Ann. Stat. 4*, 1200–1209.

Simon, R., E. Korn, L. McShane, M. Radmacher, G. Wright, and Y. Zhao (2003). *Design and Analysis of DNA Microarray Investigations*. Springer 2003.

Smith, M. and G. Glass (1977). Meta-analysis of psychotherapy outcome studies. *Am. Psychol. 32(9)*, 752–760.

Smith, S., S. Caudill, K. Steinberg, and S. Thacker (1995). On combining dose-response data from epidemiological studies by meta-analysis. *Stat Med 14*(5-7), 531–44.

Smith-Warner, S., J. Ritz, D. Hunter, and D. Albanes (2002). Dietary fat and risk of lung cancer in a pooled analysis of prospective studies. *Cancer Epidemiol Biomarkers Prev 11*, 987–92.

Spix, C., S. Schmiedel, P. Kaatsch, R. Schulze-Rath, and M. Blettner (2008). Case-Control Study on Childhood Cancer in the Vicinity of Nuclear Power Plants in Germany 1980-2003. *Eur J Cancer 44*, 275–284.

Steimer, J., S. Vozeh, A. Racine-Poon, N. Holford, and R. O'Neill (1994). The population approach: Rationale, methods, and applications in clinical pharmacology and drug development. In P. G. Welling and L. P. Balant (Eds.), *Pharmacokinetics of Drugs*, Chapter 15, pp. 404–451. Berlin, Germany: Springer-Verlag.

Stone, R. (1988). Investigations of excess environmental risks around putative sources: statistical problems and a proposed test. *Stat Med 7*(6), 649–60.

Stukel, T. (2008). Determinants of Plasma Retinol and Beta-Carotene Levels. http://lib.stat.cmu. edu/datasets/Plasma_Retinol.

Susko, E. (2003). Weighted tests of homogeneity for testing the number of components in a mixture. *Computational Statistics and Data Analysis 41*(3-4), 367–378.

Sutton, A. and J. Higgins (2008). Recent developments in meta-analysis. *Stat Med 27*(5), 625–50.

Sutton, A., D. Kendrick, and C. Coupland (2008). Meta-analysis of individual- and aggregate-level data. *Stat Med 27*(5), 651–69.

Sutton, A. J., K. R. Abram, D. R. Jones, T. A. Sheldon, and F. Song (2000). *Methods for Meta-analysis in medical research*. John Wiley and Sons, Ltd.

Swede, H., A. L. Mirand, R. J. Menezes, and K. B. Moysich (2005). Association of regular aspirin use and breast cancer risk. *Oncology 68*, 40–47.

Tango, T. (2002). Score tests for detecting excess risks around putative sources. *Stat Med. 21*, 497–514.

Tenmoto, H., M. Kudo, and M. Shimbo (2000). Selection of the number of components using a genetic algorithm for mixture model classifiers. *Advances in pattern recognition 1876*, 511–520.

Terry, M. B., M. D. Gammon, F. F. Zhang, H. Tawfik, S. L. Teitelbaum, J. A. Britton, K. Subbaramaiah, A. J. Dannenberg, and A. I. Neugut (2004, May). Association of frequency and duration of aspirin use and hormone receptor status with breast cancer risk. *JAMA 291*, 2433–2440.

Thode, H. C., S. J. Finch, and N. R. Mendell (1988). Simulated percentage points for the null distribution of the likelihood ratio test for a mixture of two normals. *Biometrics 44*(4), 1195–1201.

Thompson, S. (1994). Why sources of heterogeneity in meta-analysis should be investigated. *BMJ 309*, 1351–1355.

Thompson, S. and S. Sharp (1999). Explaining heterogeneity in meta-analysis: a comparison of methods. *Stat Med. 18*, 2693–708.

Tiago de Oliveira, J. (1965). Some elementary tests for mixtures of distributions, in Classical and Contagious Discrete Distributions (GP Patil ed.) Pergamon, New York, 379–384.

Titterington, D. M., A. Smith, and U. Makov (1985). *Statistical Analysis of Finite Mixture Distributions*. New York: Wiley.

Tjia, J., J. Colbert, and D. Back (1996). Theophylline metabolism in human liver microsomes: inhibition studies. *J Pharmacol Exp Ther 276*(3), 912–7.

Tozer, T. and M. Rowland (2006). *Introduction to Pharmacokinetics and Pharmacodynamics: The Quantitative Basis of Drug Therapy*. Lippincott Williams & Wilkins.

Ugarte, M., B. Ibanez, and A. Militino (2006). Modelling risks in disease mapping. *Stat Methods Med Res 15*(1), 21–35.

Ursin, G., M. Longenecker, R. Haile, and S. Greenland (1995). A meta-analysis of body mass index and risk of premenopausal breast cancer. *Epidemiology 6*, 137–141.

U.S. Department of Health and Human Services: Food and Drug Administration (1999, February). Guidance for industry: Population pharmacokinetics.

Vainio H, M. G. (1998). Cyclo-oxygenase 2 and breast cancer prevention. *BMJ. 317*, 828–828.

van de Vijver, M. J., Y. D. He, L. J. van't Veer, H. Dai, A. A. Hart, D. W. Voskuil, G. J. Schreiber, J. L. Peterse, C. Roberts, M. J. Marton, M. Parrish, D. Atsma, A. Witteveen, A. Glas, L. Delahaye, T. van der Velde, H. Bartelink, S. Rodenhuis, E. T. Rutgers, S. H. Friend, and R. Bernards (2002). A gene-expression signature as a predictor of survival in breast cancer. *N Engl J Med 347*(25), 1999–2009.

van Houwelingen, H., L. Arends, and T. Stijnen (2002). Advanced methods in meta-analyis: multivariate approach and meta-regression. *Statistics in Medicine 59*, 589–624.

van Houwelingen, H. C., T. Bruinsma, A. A. Hart, L. J. Van't Veer, and L. F. Wessels (2006). Cross-validated Cox regression on microarray gene expression data. *Stat Med 25*(18), 3201–16.

van't Veer, L. J., H. Y. Dai, M. J. van de Vijver, Y. D. D. He, A. A. M. Hart, M. Mao, H. L. Peterse, K. van der Kooy, M. J. Marton, A. T. Witteveen, G. J. Schreiber, R. M. Kerkhoven, C. Roberts, P. S. Linsley, R. Bernards, and S. H. Friend (2002). Gene expression profiling predicts clinical outcome of breast cancer. *Nature 415*(6871), 530–536.

van't Veer, L. J., S. Paik, and D. F. Hayes (2005). Gene expression profiling of breast cancer: a new tumor marker. *J Clin Oncol 23*(8), 1631–5.

Venables, W. and B. Ripley (2002). *Modern applied statistics with S. 4th ed.* Statistics and Computing. New York, NY: Springer. xi, 495 p.

Verbeek, J. J., J. R. J. Nunnink, and N. Vlassis (2006). Accelerated EM-based clustering of large data sets. *Data Mining and Knowledge Discovery 13*(3), 291–307.

Viechtbauer, W. (2006). MiMa an S-plus/R function to fit meta-analytic mixed-, random-, and fixed-effects models [computer software and manual]. Retrieved from http://www.wvbauer.com/.

Viele, K. and B. Tong (2002). Modeling with mixtures of linear regressions. *Statistics and Computing 12*(4), 315–330.

Vlassis, N. and A. Likas (2002). A greedy EM algorithm for Gaussian mixture learning. *Neural Processing Letters 15*(1), 77–87.

Wahrendorf, J., G. Mahon, and M. Schumacher (1985). A nonparametric approach to the statistical analysis of mutagenicity data. *Mutat Res 147*(1-2), 5–13.

Waller, L., B. Turnbull, L. Clark, and P. Nasca (1992). Chronic disease surveillance and testing of clustering of disease and exposure - application to leukemia incidence and TCE-contaminated dumpsites in upstate New-York. *Environmetrics 3*(3), 281–300.

Wang, P., M. Puterman, I. Cockburn, and N. Le (1996). Mixed Poisson regression models with covariate dependent rates. *Biometrics 52*(2), 381–400.

Watanabe, M. and K. Yamaguchi (2004). *The EM Algorithm and Related Statistical Models (Statistics, a Series of Textbooks and Monographs)*. Marcel Dekker, New York.

Wedel, M. (2002). Concomitant variables in finite mixture models. *Statistica Neerlandica 56*(3), 362–375.

Weed, D. (1997). Methodologic guidelines for review papers. *JNCI 89*, 6–7.

White, H. (1982). Maximum likehood estimation of misspecified models. *Econometrics 50*, 1–26.

Whitehead, A. (2001). *Meta-analysis of controlled clinical trials*. John Wiley and Sons, Ltd, West Sussex, England .

WHO (2002). Incidence, mortality and survival database.

Winter, M. E. (2004). *Basic Clinical Pharmacokinetics* (fourth ed.). Baltimore, MD: Lippincott Williams & Wilkins.

Wu, C.F. (1983). On the convergence properties of the EM-algorithm. *Annals of Statistics 11*(1), 95–103.

Xiang, L. and A. Lee (2005). Sensitivity of test for overdispersion in Poisson regression. *Biom J* 47(2), 167–76.

Xiang, L., K. Yau, A. Lee, and W. Fung (2005). Influence diagnostics for two-component Poisson mixture regression models: applications in public health. *Stat Med* 24(19), 3053–71.

Yasui, Y., H. Liu, J. Benach, and M. Winget (2000). An empirical evaluation of various priors in the empirical Bayes estimation of small area disease risks. *Stat Med* 19(17-18), 2409–20.

Yoon, Y., H. Park, K. Park, J. Kim, Y. Chang, and J. Song (2006). Associations between CYP2E1 promoter polymorphisms and plasma 1,3-dimethyluric acid/theophylline ratios. *Eur J Clin Pharmacol* 62(8), 627–31.

Zeeger, M., A. Jellema, and H. Ostrer (2003). Empiric risk of prostate carcinoma for relatives of patients with prostate carcinoma: a meta-analysis. *Cancer 97*, 1894–1903.

Zeiger, E. (2004). History and rationale of genetic toxicity testing: an impersonal, and sometimes personal, view. *Environ Mol Mutagen* 44(5), 363–71.

Zhang, Y., P. F. Coogan, J. R. Palmer, B. L. Strom, and L. Rosenberg (2005, Jul). Use of nonsteroidal antiinflammatory drugs and risk of breast cancer: the case-control surveillance study revisited. *Am. J. Epidemiol. 162*, 165–170.

Subject Index

Author Index